DISCARD

ENCYCLOPEDIA OF
FAMILY HEALTH

—————— THIRD EDITION ——————

ENCYCLOPEDIA OF
FAMILY HEALTH

—— THIRD EDITION ——

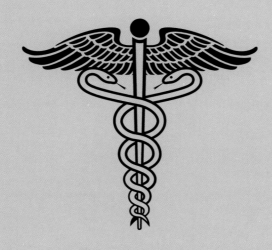

CONSULTANTS

David B. Jacoby, M.D.
Johns Hopkins School of Medicine

Robert M. Youngson, M.D.
Royal Society of Medicine

VOLUME 12

PIGEON CHEST — PSYCHOSOMATIC PROBLEMS

MARSHALL CAVENDISH
New York · London · Singapore

MEDICAL CONSULTANTS

Second Edition
David B. Jacoby, M.D.
Johns Hopkins School of Medicine
Associate Professor of Pulmonary and Critical
  Care Medicine

Third Edition
Robert M. Youngson, M.D.
Fellow of the Royal Society of Medicine
Officer of the Order of St John of Jerusalem
Diploma in Tropical Medicine and Hygiene
Fellow of the Royal College of Ophthalmologists

CONTRIBUTORS TO THIRD EDITION

David Arnot   Tom Jackson
Deborah Evans   Nathan Lepora
Leon Gray   Fiona Plowman
Joanna Griffin   Alison Tarrant
Tim Harris   Aruna Vasudevan
John Jackson

Picture Credits
(b – bottom; t – top; r – right; l – left; c – center)

Cover: Dynamic Graphics: John Foxx & Images 4 Communication b/l, b/r; PhotoDisc: Don Farrall b/c, Keith Brofsky c, t/r.

Alan Hutchinson Library: 1607t; Anthea Sieveking: 1676, 1677all, 1679all; ARS: Keith Weller 1701b; Aspect: Fiona Nichols 1638st; Biophoto Associates: 1598, 1599, 1605t/l, 1691t/c; Bruce Coleman Ltd: Charles Henneghien 1633; Bubbles Photo Library: 1657all; C James Webb: 1607b/l, 1607b/r; Camera Press: 1639b; Camilla Jessel: 1686; Clarks: 1684; Colegate: 1608all, 1609t/l, 1609t/r; Colorific: 1707, C Bevlaque 1605t/r, Claus C Mayer 1663b, Linda Bartlett 1621c, Wayne Source 1713; Corbis: Bettmann 1606, Charles Gupton 1719, Chris Jones 1705, Dan Lamont 1693, Erik Freeland 1641b, John Henley 1724b, Jose Luis Pelaez Inc 1597t, Leif Skoogfors 1634, Lester Lefkowitz 1698, Lester V Bergman 1706, Norbert Schaefer 1594; Dr Zeegan: 1643; Getty Images: 1597b, 1621t, 1656, 1661, 1662t/l, 1681t/l, Bruce Ayres 1714, Janeart Inc 1601b, Jim Jordan 1717b, Jon Gray 1649, Marc Grimberg 1715b, Owen Franken 1650; Hemera: 1701t; Ingram Publishing: 1701b; J Allan Cash: 1641t; John Watney: 1623b; Magnum: George Roger 1619; Max Rendall FRCS: 1645, 1670; Mary Evans Picture Library: 1711all; N Shah FRCS: 1699b; National Library of Medicine: 1722; Oxford Scientific Films: Newfried/Okapia 1708; Paul Beviti: 1631; Paul Windson: 1683, 1688all; PHIL: Dr Mae Melvin 1704, Jim Gathany 1703; PhotoDisc: Alex L Fradkin 1639t, Dan Farrall 1682b, Keith Brofsky 1602, 1610t/r, 1659, 1680, Sami Sarkis 1640b, Skipp Nall 1603, Steve Mason 1672, Suza Scalora 1685t/l; Photos.com: 1637t/r; Queen Victoria Hospital, Sussex: 1612all; Rex Features: 1640t, 1655, 1717t, AGB Photo Agency 1724t, AIRO 1616t, Alexander Caminada 1723, Ann Pickford 1651, Fotex Medien Agentur GMBH 1673, IPC Magazines/Chat 1648, 1654, Isopress 1632, Lehtikuva Oy 1721, Phanie Agency 1671, 1675, 1682c, 1709, Stewart Cook 1674, Sutton-Hibbert 1720, Wil Blanche 1725; Robert Harding: 1635t/l, 1690; Roger Payling 1658all, 1710; Ron Sutherland: 1692; Sally Greenhill: 1689; Spectrum: 1613; Science Photo Library: 1623t/l, 1623t, 1624b, 1691t/r, BSIP LECA 1611, Damien Lovegrove 1628, Dr P Marazzi 1626, 1627, Francoise Sauze 1610t/l, 1715t, Hank Morgan 1644, 1646, Hattie Young 1609b, J C Revy 1620, James Stevenson 1699t, Klaus Guldbrandsen 1668, Omikron 1635t/r, Peter Menzel 1696, Peter Ryan 1667, Publiphoto Diffusion 1669, Tim Beddow 1630; St Mary's Hospital School: AVC Department 1601; Topham Picturepoint: Rommel Pecson/ The Image Works 1691b; US Customs: James Tourtellotte 1652; Vision International: Anthea Sieveking 1666, 1681c, 1681b, CNRI 1691t/l, Paolo Koch 1637t/l, 1638b, 1681t/r, 1718; Wellcome Photo Library: 1590, 1592, 1593; Zefa: 1595, 1624t, 1647, 1660, 1663t, 1682t, 1716.

Marshall Cavendish
99 White Plains Road
Tarrytown, NY 10591-9001

www.marshallcavendish.com

© 2005, 1998, 1991 Marshall Cavendish Corporation

All rights reserved. No part of this book may be reproduced or utilized in any form or by any means, electronic or mechanical, including photo-copying, recording, or by any information storage and retrieval system, without prior written permission from the publisher and copyright holder.

Library of Congress Cataloging-in-Publication Data

Encyclopedia of family health / David B. Jacoby, Robert M. Youngson.--
3rd ed.
    p. cm.
Includes bibliographical references and index.
  ISBN 0-7614-7486-2 (set)
  ISBN 0-7614-7498-6 (vol 12)
1. Medicine, Popular--Encyclopedias. 2. Health--Encyclopedias. 1. Jacoby, David B. II. Youngson, R. M. III. Marshall Cavendish Corporation. IV. Title
RC81.A2E5 2004
610'.3--dc22   2003065554

Printed in China
08 07 06 05 04 5 4 3 2 1

Marshall Cavendish

Editor: Joyce Tavolacci
Editorial Director: Paul Bernabeo
Production Manager: Alan Tsai

The Brown Reference Group

Project Editor: Anne Hildyard
Editors: Jane Lanigan, Sally McFall
Designers: Jeni Child, Reg Cox, Karen Frazer
Picture Researcher: Clare Newman
Indexer: Kay Ollerenshaw
Illustrations: Samantha J. Elmhurst
Managing Editor: Tim Cooke
Art Director: Dave Goodman

CONTENTS

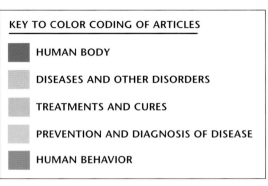

KEY TO COLOR CODING OF ARTICLES

HUMAN BODY

DISEASES AND OTHER DISORDERS

TREATMENTS AND CURES

PREVENTION AND DIAGNOSIS OF DISEASE

HUMAN BEHAVIOR

Pigeon chest

Questions and Answers

My daughter has a pigeon chest that was brought about by asthma. A friend told me that she would improve if we moved to a rural area. What do you advise?

While there is some evidence that asthma and pigeon chest are helped by breathing clean air, there is no certainty that this will be the case. The move away from familiar surroundings and friends may upset your daughter, and could even make the problem worse. You should think carefully before moving. In the meantime your daughter should get involved in lots of outdoor activities. The exercise and companionship may be more beneficial than uprooting the entire family.

Is it possible for a baby to be born with pigeon chest?

This happens very rarely. More often the deformity is noticed as a child grows up. Usually pigeon chest has no specific cause, but it may sometimes be caused by a respiratory disease.

Can pigeon chest be passed on from one generation to the next?

There is no evidence for this, although there may be a family tendency toward respiratory complaints, such as asthma, that may bring about the deformity.

Does pigeon chest need treatment?

Pigeon chest is almost always harmless. However, when it is caused by a respiratory disease, such as asthma, it indicates that the asthma is not being treated adequately. Modern treatments are usually able to control asthma well, so that the condition rarely causes pigeon chest.
   Occasionally, when a child's chest is badly deformed, corrective surgery may be considered.

In a condition known as pigeon chest, a person's sternum, or breastbone, may be slightly deformed, making the breast bow outward. It may develop as a result of respiratory illness, but more often develops for no particular reason.

Pigeon chest, or pigeon breast, is the name used to describe an abnormal prominence of the breastbone. This bone, located in the center of the chest at the front of the body, is known anatomically as the sternum. Some of the ribs are connected to the sternum. In pigeon chest, which is more common in children than in adults, the breastbone is curved outward, giving the chest a birdlike look. Occasionally, babies are born with pigeon chest, but it is more likely to develop spontaneously during childhood. The condition can also develop as a result of illnesses that affect breathing.

Structure of the breastbone

Pigeon chest can develop because of the way in which the breastbone is constructed. Like the rest of the skeleton, the sternum in a fetus starts out as a gristly substance known as cartilage. When fully formed, the sternum consists of a row of five bones, and a tailpiece called the xiphoid process. Between these bones are large disks of cartilage; this cartilage does not become fully hardened—by being impregnated with bone—until people reach the age of about 40.
   In children, the five main bones of the sternum, and the cartilage connections between them, are extremely elastic. It is not until after the age of 25 or so that the cartilage starts to be invaded by bone. In fact it is not uncommon for the cartilage between the two topmost bones to remain

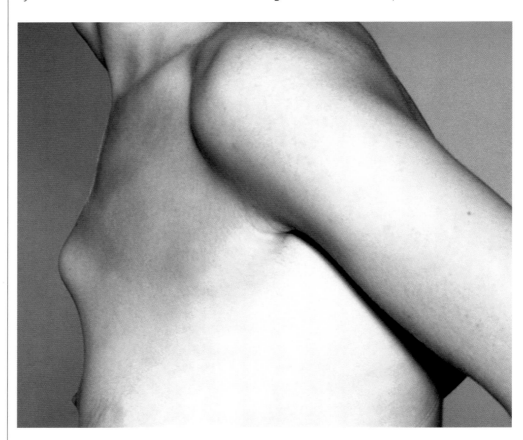

▲ *Although pigeon chest usually becomes less noticeable as a person grows older, the outward curve of this girl's sternum (breastbone) can still be seen clearly.*

STRUCTURE OF STERNUM (BREASTBONE) AND RIBS IN MIDDLE AGE

**STERNUM
BEFORE BIRTH**

**STERNUM
AT PUBERTY**

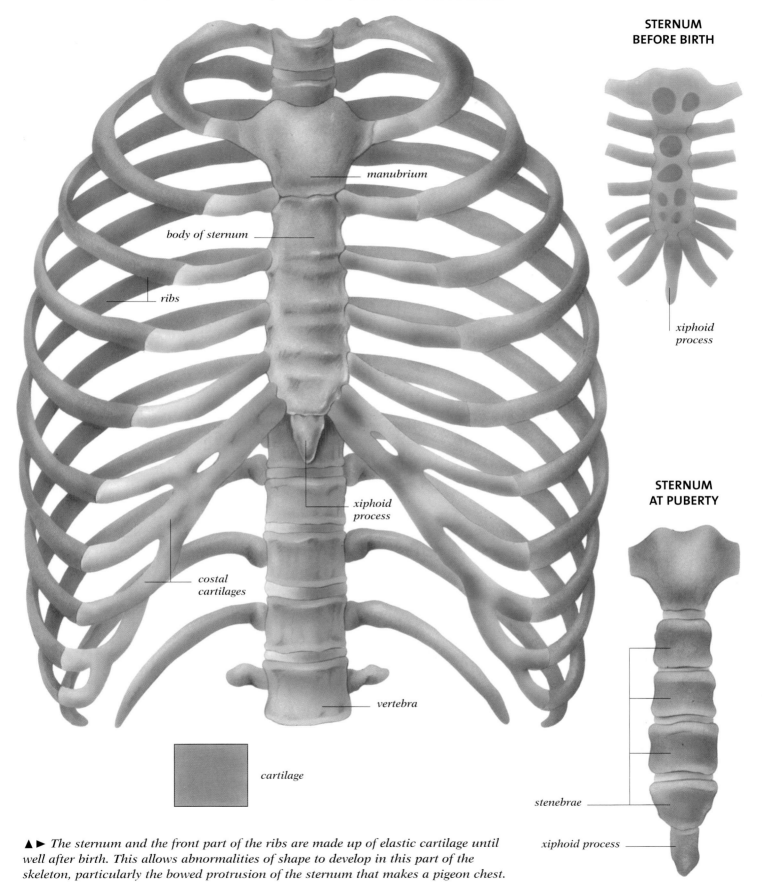

manubrium

body of sternum

ribs

xiphoid
process

costal
cartilages

vertebra

xiphoid
process

stenebrae

xiphoid process

cartilage

▲ ▶ *The sternum and the front part of the ribs are made up of elastic cartilage until well after birth. This allows abnormalities of shape to develop in this part of the skeleton, particularly the bowed protrusion of the sternum that makes a pigeon chest.*

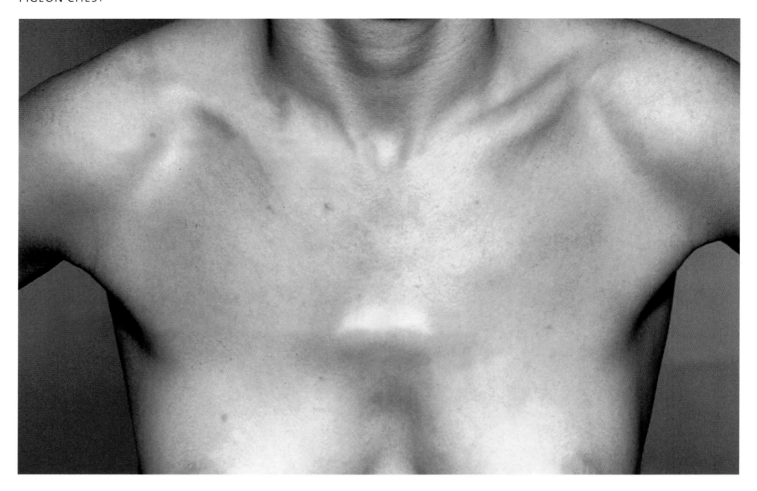

▲ *Excessive deep breathing, the result of a respiratory illness such as tuberculosis, asthma, or cystic fibrosis, will occasionally cause pigeon chest to develop.*

as cartilage for the whole of a person's life. The reason for this elasticity is that some movement is essential to allow the chest to expand every time people breathe air into their lungs.

How pigeon chest develops

Sometimes the bones of the sternum are laid down in a slightly abnormal fashion, making the breast bow outward. There is usually no underlying reason for the deformity in such cases. However, a less common cause of pigeon chest is excessive deep breathing over a long period of time. This causes air to become trapped in the lungs; that condition in turn has the effect of stretching the cartilage connections abnormally and causing overactivity of the chest muscles. Tuberculosis used to be a significant cause of this excessively deep breathing (see Tuberculosis). Now that tuberculosis is not the problem it once was in the West, the conditions that are most likely to cause pigeon chest in a child are asthma and cystic fibrosis.

In adults who have asthma or bronchitis, the airways into and out of the lungs become abnormally narrow, and this narrowing tends to allow air to accumulate within the lungs (see Bronchitis). The body's natural reaction is to take deeper breaths, usually through the mouth, to get enough air into the lungs. The deep breathing tends to make matters worse, in that the trapping of excess air in the lungs becomes even more exaggerated.

What should be done

If parents are worried that their child's chest is beginning to take on a pigeonlike appearance, it is important that they take him or her to a doctor for a thorough checkup. This will probably involve a chest X ray. The doctor will first determine whether there is an underlying cause of the pigeon chest. If there is, the doctor will treat it, and this will help the chest to return to its normal shape. In such cases, the child will probably not suffer any permanent deformity.

In most childhood cases of pigeon chest when there is deformity for no particular reason, this should cause no physical problems— the child will probably have normal breathing and respiration. In the rare cases when pigeon chest is caused by asthma that has been treated inadequately, correct treatment of that underlying condition will halt any further development of the deformity.

In most cases of pigeon chest, the condition causes problems only when a child becomes embarrassed or upset by the appearance of his or her chest. If this is beginning to cause the child severe psychological problems, a doctor may consider corrective cosmetic surgery. However, this type of surgery on pigeon chest is extremely unusual. Instead, a child may be helped to overcome his or her embarrassment if adults reassure him or her that a pigeon chest usually becomes less noticeable as a person gets older. Men tend to develop broad shoulders that disguise the irregularity of the chest, and in women breast tissue will often mask the condition.

See also: **Asthma; Cartilage; Cystic fibrosis; Skeleton**

Pigeon toes

Questions and Answers

My daughter is 18 months old and is about to have a checkup at the health clinic. Should I mention her pigeon toes to the doctor?

Yes. It is always advisable to tell the doctor about any concerns. The doctor will check your daughter's legs and feet and the way she walks. You will be advised to see your family doctor or a specialist only if the pigeon toes seem severe, or if one leg is affected more than the other.

My eight-year-old son has pigeon toes. Both he and my husband walk with their kneecaps facing inward slightly. Do you think my son's condition will improve?

It may improve, but this is less likely after six or seven years of age, and if pigeon toes run in the family. If your son does not have difficulty walking, there is nothing to worry about. Many athletic people are slightly pigeon-toed.

My 12-month-old son has taken his first solo steps, but he stands with his toes turned inward. Does he need treatment?

Many toddlers turn their toes inward when they start to walk; this position helps them to balance. It usually corrects itself by the time the child is three or four years old, and no treatment is needed.

My husband enjoys sports, and is worried that our son's pigeon toes will interfere with his ability to do well in athletics. Is this likely?

No. Orthopedic surgeons assure us that the condition, even if it is fairly obvious, is highly unlikely to limit athletic prowess. In theory, only a severe degree of toeing in might cause a problem. You should check out all the successful sportspeople who show toeing in.

Many parents worry unnecessarily about their child's pigeon toes. The condition does not affect walking or running, and usually corrects itself over time. Even when it does persist, it can be treated successfully.

"Pigeon toes" is a term used generally when the toes of both feet turn inward. The problem, which is also called "toeing in," can arise from a number of different causes. However, the exact cause of the condition may be regarded as fairly unimportant, because in almost all affected children toeing in corrects itself naturally with growth.

Femoral anteversion

The most common type of toeing in is femoral anteversion. In this case, the affected individual —who is usually a child—walks with the whole of his or her leg turned inward from the hip. The kneecaps tend to point toward each other instead of forward. This is because there is actual inward rotation of the thighbone (femur) at the ball-and-socket hip joint, and consequently of the whole of the leg. In such cases the result is some, usually minor, reduction in the affected child's ability to rotate the thigh outward. Although his or her gait may appear a little clumsy, little or no disability is caused. Indeed, as the child grows, the degree of toeing in will gradually become less and less prominent.

The natural progress of femoral anteversion is for the femur to gradually rotate outward until the child reaches the age of about eight; then there is a slower increase in the power of outward rotation until he or she reaches age 15 or 16. Research has shown that little is to be achieved by special shoes, splints, or leg braces in such cases.

Children who show this common form of toeing in often prefer to watch television or read a book sitting on the floor with the knees facing each other and their lower legs flat on the ground pointing outward. This is because in this position the thighbones are rotated fully inward; this position is more comfortable for children with the condition. However, to improve the ability to rotate the thigh outward, it is best if such children are encouraged to sit on the floor in a partial lotus or Buddha position with the knees outward and the legs crossed (see Yoga), especially while watching TV. This position ensures full outward rotation of the thighs. Parents might insist that watching TV is allowed only if the child adopts and maintains this cross-legged position.

In older children, it may also be helpful for parents to encourage more athletic activities, such as skating or ballet dancing, in which the external rotation of the legs is necessary. The child's ambition to be successful in either of these or other athletic pursuits may provide sufficient motivation to cure the condition.

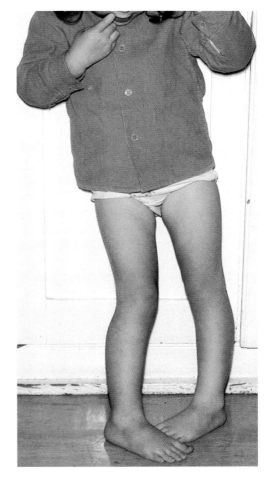

▶ *A pigeon-toed child may appear a little clumsy, but he or she suffers no disability and soon grows out of the condition.*

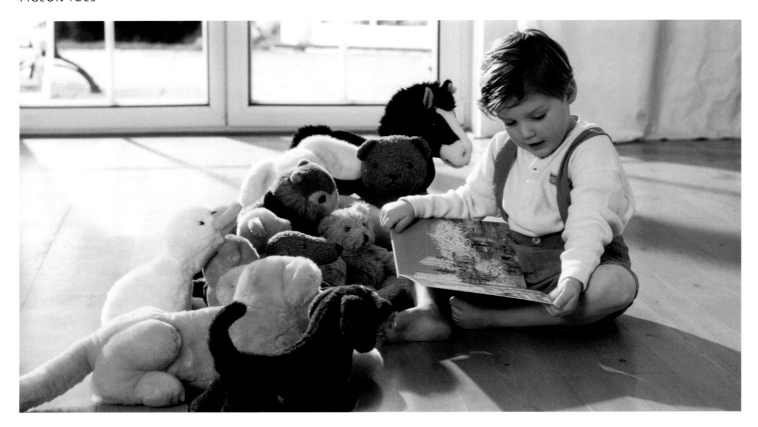

▲ *Encouraging a child who has pigeon toes to sit with his or her knees apart should improve the condition.*

The appearance of pigeon toes can also result because a child's forefeet were turned inward (metatarsus varus) at birth. This problem becomes much more noticeable when the child is learning to walk. In such cases, although the forefeet turn inward, other parts of the limb remain normal and the knees face forward.

Confusion with clubfoot

Metatarsus varus is not a form of clubfoot, and should not be confused with this much more serious condition. Clubfoot, also known as talipes equinovarus, is present from birth and is characterized by undue straightening at the ankle with turning in of both the heel and the sole of the foot. It usually affects one side only. Talipes tends to run in families and affects about one baby in 1,000.

The implications of clubfoot are much more serious than those of toeing in, and it is important that medical treatment should not be delayed because of any confusion between the two conditions. Pigeon toes can be corrected temporarily by holding the knee and rotating the child's whole leg outward. However, in talipes, parents will notice that this maneuver does not alter the position of the foot. If they suspect that their child may have talipes, parents should seek medical advice immediately. In some cases, talipes is accompanied by other orthopedic problems, and early examination is required.

Talipes equinovarus indicates a shortening of tissues and requires manipulation from birth, or as soon as possible after birth. This treatment would be followed by splinting to maintain the correct position of the foot. The earlier such treatment is applied, the more successful it will be. In cases of delay, the foot will become rigid in a matter of days and more invasive treatment may be required. About half of the children who are born with clubfoot require later surgery to lengthen soft tissue structures that have become contracted.

Treatment

In clear cases of pigeon toes it is seldom necessary to take the matter any further than has been already described. However, in unusual cases when the condition persists, correction is possible using plaster casts and, occasionally, surgery.

Some children have femoral anteversion, a turning in of the whole leg; usually, this condition resolves itself by age eight. In the past some children with this type of toeing in were given leg splints or special shoes to wear. However, these are no longer used, because it has been found that they can be harmful.

In the few cases in which the condition does not resolve itself over time, walking or running is not normally impaired. However, there may still be concern because of the child's appearance, which may cause him or her to be self-conscious or embarrassed. The only effective method of correction in this case involves an operation to realign the bones of the upper leg so that the feet face forward. This is a major procedure, but it is rarely necessary. It is never performed before the age of eight and should be considered only in cases in which the child has no external rotation of the leg beyond the neutral position. The operation is called an osteotomy and it involves cutting through both thighbones, rotating the lower ends outward, and then treating both legs in much the same way as if the child had suffered fractures in both legs. The healing of fractures is fairly rapid in children of this age and good results are likely. However, as in all surgical procedures, complications are always a possibility.

See also: **Clubfoot; Feet; Fractures; Orthopedics**

Pins and needles

Questions and Answers

When I went camping recently I slept on the ground and often woke up with pins and needles in my leg. Should I be worried?

Probably not. It is likely that sleeping on the ground meant that pressure was put on a peripheral nerve in your thigh, causing some of the nerve fibers to work less well. Pins and needles are your body's way of telling you to relieve the pressure. If the prickly feeling clears quickly after changing position, there is nothing to worry about. If the sensation persists, you should see a doctor.

Once, after I had received some bad news, I noticed that I was breathing quickly and had pins and needles around my mouth. What caused this?

Fast breathing, or hyperventilation, occurs in some people when they are upset. Hyperventilation causes an abnormal loss of carbon dioxide, a change in blood acidity, and a consequent drop in blood calcium. Nerves require calcium ion movement for proper function, and this is why your nerves were affected.

I often get pins and needles near my little finger and along the outside of my hand. Is this something to be worried about?

It may be that one of the nerves to the hand, the ulnar nerve, is getting trapped in its journey around the bony part of the elbow. People who suffer from this may need surgery to free the nerve at the elbow. Some jobs involve unusual amounts of pressure on the elbows, so it may be worth looking at your regular activities to see if this is what is happening. If you work in an office, for example, you may be resting your elbows on your desk for prolonged periods of time, and this could be what is causing the pins and needles.

The feeling of "pins and needles" usually acts as a warning that pressure is being put on a nerve, so is an important part of the body's defense against damage. However, the sensation is also sometimes a symptom of disease.

Most people have experienced "pins and needles" at one time or another. It is the prickly feeling that an individual gets when one of his or her limbs has "gone to sleep"—or gone numb—after a long time in a cramped position, and normal sensation is just beginning to return.

Although it is most often felt in everyday situations, the same or a similar sensation can also be part of some diseases—especially those diseases that involve the peripheral nerves. Abnormalities of the brain and spinal cord can also cause pins and needles when those areas that analyze the messages coming from the nerves are damaged. In these more serious cases, however, the prickly feeling of pins and needles may not go away, and may be accompanied by other symptoms, depending on the particular cause. Such a combination helps doctors to distinguish this type of symptomatic pins and needles from the much more common and harmless sensation that people experience from time to time.

Causes of simple pins and needles

The most common cause of pins and needles is pressure on the peripheral nerves. When a person's legs and arms feel normal, they do so because his or her brain is getting messages

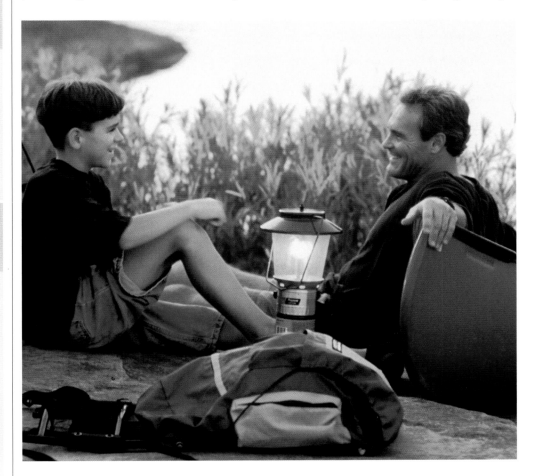

▲ *Sleeping or sitting on a hard surface can cause unusual pressure on the peripheral nerves. Pins and needles tell a person to move the affected limb.*

Are pins and needles always due to pressure on the nerve in the area in which they are felt?

No, although this is the most common cause. There are certain diseases in which pins and needles are symptomatic and may occur in various parts of the body. These are usually conditions involving a generalized inflammation of part of the nervous system. Such disorders include diabetes, multiple sclerosis, alcoholism, and syphilis. If there is no local cause for a patient's pins and needles, the doctor will carry out tests to see if one of these general causes is present. In such cases, the pins and needles do not disappear when the patient changes position.

Is it true that circulatory disorders can cause pins and needles?

Yes. As well as pressure, any other factor that disturbs the normal functioning of the sensory nerves may cause pins and needles. Therefore, if for any reason blood circulation in any part of the body is poor—for example, in cold weather or if a person is suffering from chilblains (a swelling or sore caused by exposure to cold)—and the nerves do not get sufficient oxygen to work normally, some numbness or pins and needles may be felt.

I sometimes wake up with pins and needles all down one arm and am terrified that I am developing multiple sclerosis. Is this at all likely?

Almost certainly not. First, multiple sclerosis does not give rise to the symptoms you describe. Second, there is a simpler and much more probable explanation: that you sleep in a position that leads to pressure being put on the nerve trunk that supplies the part of your arm in which you get the pins and needles. It is only if the pins and needles fail to disappear when you get up that you need to worry about the possibility of a more serious condition.

constantly from many different nerves in the limbs and—using all of this information—is forming a picture of what is going on in those limbs. The nerves that are involved in sending the information for this picture are varied in type and size; as a result, they differ in how they respond to any damage, however slight that damage may be.

For example, when a person's legs are crossed for a long time, the nerve to the foot—which is close to the surface at the inside of the knee—sustains pressure from the leg underneath it, and some of the nerve fibers work less well. Since there are different types of nerves, they respond quite differently to one another in response to this pressure. Thus the spinal cord cells and those of the thalamus in the brain, which carry out sophisticated analysis of the incoming messages, start getting an incorrect combination of messages. As a result, the sensations that the spinal cord and the thalamus relay to the person's conscious brain are also jumbled. The nerves that convey messages of pricking and pinpoint pain transmit messages more effectively than the other nerves. The pins-and-needles sensation that they convey, therefore, tends to be the only one felt by the person.

In addition to the nerves to the upper surface of the foot, other common sites for nerves to be pressed on are in the arm and in the thigh.

HOW PINS AND NEEDLES CAN BE CAUSED

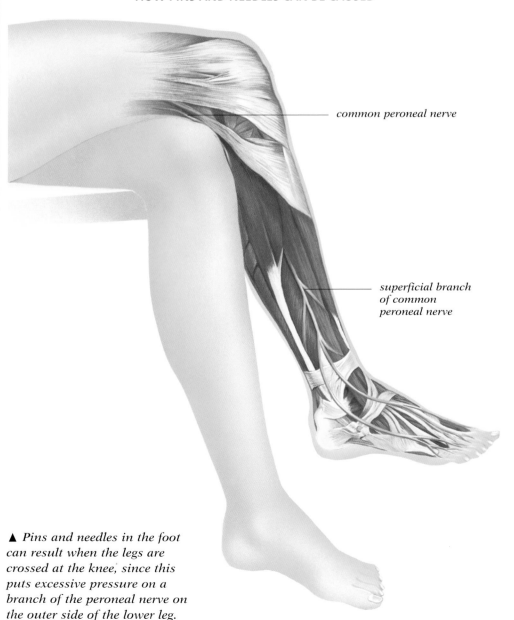

common peroneal nerve

superficial branch of common peroneal nerve

▲ *Pins and needles in the foot can result when the legs are crossed at the knee, since this puts excessive pressure on a branch of the peroneal nerve on the outer side of the lower leg.*

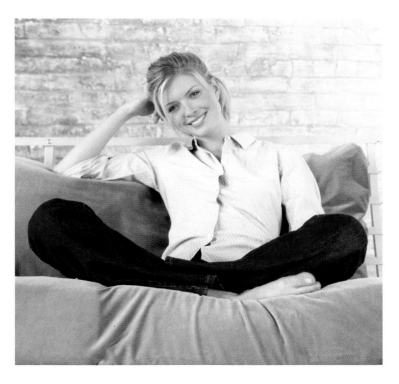

▲ *Sitting cross-legged may be comfortable for a time, but could eventually put pressure on a nerve, causing pins and needles.*

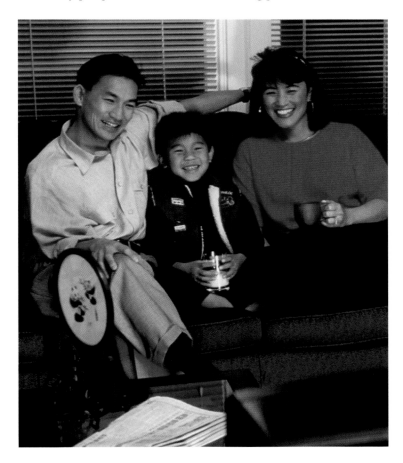

▲ *If the sensation of pins and needles persists after a person uncrosses his or her legs, medical advice should be sought.*

The everyday sensation of pins and needles has a purpose: it usually stimulates the person in question to move his or her affected limb into a more comfortable position before serious harm can be done to the nerve involved (see Pain).

Diseases of the nerves

Pins and needles can also be caused by one of a number of disorders of the nerves. Such disorders may occur as a result of inflammation of the nerves, damage from poisons (including alcohol), diabetes, or—more rarely—a remote effect of a cancer elsewhere in the body.

The feeling of pins and needles is experienced because the disorder tends to disturb the function of different types of nerve fibers to varying degrees, causing the brain to receive conflicting messages. Usually such diseases cause damage to many nerves, and the pins and needles are felt by the affected person in both feet or in all four limbs. Symptomatic pins and needles do not disappear when the person moves about or changes position.

Other damage can result from pressure on a nerve that is being exerted by nearby bones or other structures. This occurs commonly in the wrist when the median nerve is compressed as it passes through the tunnel made by bones and ligaments. The result is pins and needles in the hands, occurring usually in the middle of the night or when the hands are being used when sewing or doing other intricate handwork. This common condition, known as carpal tunnel syndrome, can be treated easily either by splinting the wrist or by surgery to relieve the pressure (see Carpal Tunnel Syndrome).

Circulation problems

Poor blood supply can slightly damage some of the fibers of a nerve and cause pins and needles in the same way as pressure.

A different cause lies behind the pins and needles in the left arm, which may occur when people suffer the extreme pain of angina or of a heart attack. In these cases, the area of the spinal cord that analyzes messages from the heart becomes highly activated. The messages of pain from the heart are so intense that they spill over and the brain interprets this as affecting the arm as well. The result is pins and needles.

Warning signs

Getting pins and needles in a leg when it has been crossed over the other leg for some time is commonplace and—if the leg recovers quickly and in the usual way—is not a cause for concern. Some of the muscles in the leg may be weak for a short time when the legs are eventually uncrossed, but the sensation will also pass quickly.

However, in general, if the sensation of pins and needles persists for long periods of time or occurs regularly in both feet and arms, then a visit to the doctor is advisable. Most people will notice such unusual features, which may act as a warning of a more serious condition. Many of the disorders of the nerves that cause pins and needles can be treated successfully, and it is reassuring for people to seek medical advice.

See also: **Brain; Circulatory system; Diabetes; Heart attack; Nervous system; Numbness; Poisoning; Spinal cord**

Pituitary gland

Questions and Answers

I heard of a woman who started to lactate when she had not had a baby. Could this have been due to a problem in her pituitary gland?

Yes. One fairly common pituitary problem is the secretion of excessive amounts of a hormone called prolactin, and this stimulates milk production. The cause is a slow-growing tumor in the gland called a prolactinoma. This can damage vision and may be fatal.

If the pituitary failed, would all the other glands also stop working?

No. The main glands affected would be the adrenal, thyroid, and sex glands. The pancreas would continue to produce insulin, and the parathyroid glands would continue to control the level of calcium. Important hormones from other glands, such as renin from the kidneys (one of the hormones concerned with retaining adequate amounts of salt and water in the body) would still be secreted.

Does your libido decline if your pituitary gland stops working?

Yes, if the condition is not treated. One of the main functions of the pituitary is to stimulate the production of sex hormones. These come from the ovaries and (to a lesser extent) from the adrenal glands in women and from the testes and adrenal glands in men. However, these hormones can be replaced if the pituitary fails.

Is the pituitary essential to life?

Yes. Pituitary failure is dangerous mainly because the adrenal glands depend on it to function. A lack of adrenal hormones, such as cortisone, is fatal. If the pituitary fails, the thyroid gland will also stop working; this too can be fatal, but replacement thyroid and cortisone can be given.

The pituitary is the main gland in the body's hormone system. Although it weighs only a few ounces, it is responsible for the control of many hormones, including those of the adrenal glands, thyroid glands, and sex glands.

The pituitary gland is found in the base of the brain. It is joined by a stalk of nervous tissue to the hypothalamus, and works closely with this part of the brain. Together, the pituitary and the hypothalamus control many aspects of the body's metabolism—the chemical processes that keep the body functioning (see Metabolism).

Structure and function

The pituitary sits inside a protective bony saddle called the sella turcica—Latin for "Turkish saddle." The sella turcica, or sella, as doctors call it, can be seen clearly on an X ray of the skull; an enlarged sella is an indication that something is wrong with the pituitary gland.

The gland itself is divided into two totally separate halves. The rear half, or posterior pituitary, is linked to the hypothalamus through the pituitary stalk. It is concerned with the production of two major hormones that are produced in the hypothalamus. From there, the two hormones travel along specialized nerve cells to the posterior pituitary. They are released from the posterior pituitary when the hypothalamus receives appropriate messages about the state of the body.

The front half of the pituitary, the anterior pituitary, produces the hormones that activate other important glands in the body; it also produces two important hormones that act on the tissues directly. The anterior pituitary is not linked to the hypothalamus directly, but it is bound closely to this part of the brain in the way that it functions.

Since the anterior pituitary has no direct nerve paths to link it with the hypothalamus, it has to depend on a series of special releasing and inhibiting factors to control hormone release. Some of these factors are themselves specialized hormones, which are released by the hypothalamus and act on the pituitary gland. The specialized hormones are carried in a set of

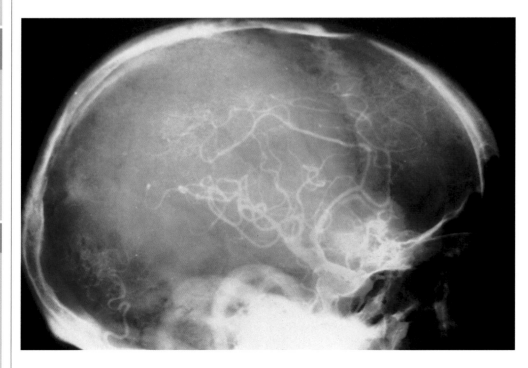

▲ *This X ray of the skull shows a tumor near the pituitary fossa, a hollow in the sella turcica. Such growths often prevent the pituitary from producing hormones normally.*

LOCATION AND STRUCTURE OF THE PITUITARY GLAND

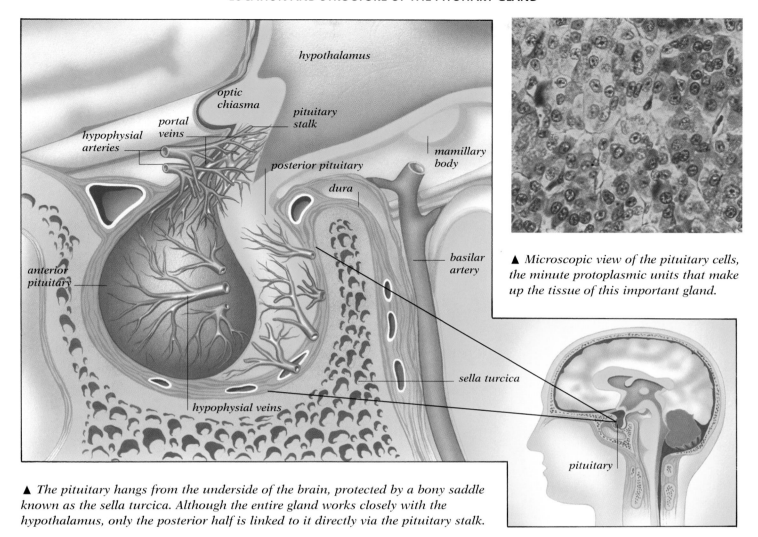

▲ *Microscopic view of the pituitary cells, the minute protoplasmic units that make up the tissue of this important gland.*

▲ *The pituitary hangs from the underside of the brain, protected by a bony saddle known as the sella turcica. Although the entire gland works closely with the hypothalamus, only the posterior half is linked to it directly via the pituitary stalk.*

blood vessels—known as the pituitary portal system—between the hypothalamus and the pituitary.

Although many of the instructions to release hormones come from the hypothalamus, the anterior pituitary also has independent control. In addition, the release of some of its secretions is inhibited by substances circulating in the bloodstream. One such secretion is the hormone TSH (thyroid-stimulating hormone), which stimulates the thyroid gland to produce its hormones. The release of TSH by the pituitary is inhibited when there are high levels of thyroid hormone already in the blood. Called negative feedback, this is an important principle in the control of many pituitary hormones.

This principle means that levels of hormones produced in glands that are far removed from the pituitary cannot rise too high; if hormone levels are already quite high, negative feedback acts on the pituitary and turns off the production of stimulating hormones.

Hormones of the pituitary

The posterior pituitary produces two hormones—antidiuretic hormone (ADH) and oxytocin. ADH is concerned with the control of water in the body. It acts on the tubules of the kidneys, so that the kidney tissue is able to withdraw more or less water (as necessary) out of the urine as it leaves the tubule. When ADH is secreted into

the blood, the kidneys tend to conserve water. When the hormone is not secreted, more water is lost in the urine (see Kidneys and Kidney Diseases). Alcohol stops the pituitary from secreting ADH; for this reason, drinking alcohol causes urination.

The role of oxytocin is less clear, but in women it is concerned with starting labor and causing the uterus to contract. It also plays an important part in starting the secretion of milk from the breasts during lactation. In males, oxytocin may be concerned with generating an orgasm.

The anterior pituitary produces six main hormones. Four of these are concerned with the control of other important glands in the body—the thyroid gland; the adrenal glands; and the gonads (the testes in the male; the ovaries in the female). The activity of the thyroid gland is triggered by TSH; the cortex (outer part) of the adrenal gland is affected by the hormone ACTH (adrenocorticotropic hormone). The overall levels of thyroid hormone and cortisone from the adrenal glands are maintained by a combination of negative feedback, which acts on the pituitary, and extra signals that come from the hypothalamus—in times of stress, for example.

The anterior pituitary also releases the hormones FSH (follicle-stimulating hormone), and LH (luteinizing hormone). These are known as gonadotropins, which are hormones that affect the sex

HORMONAL ACTIVITY OF THE PITUITARY

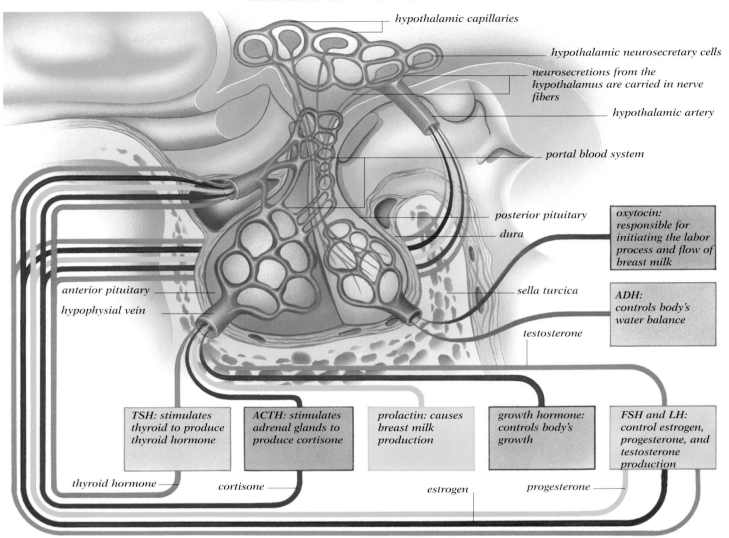

hypothalamic capillaries

hypothalamic neurosecretary cells

neurosecretions from the hypothalamus are carried in nerve fibers

hypothalamic artery

portal blood system

posterior pituitary

dura

oxytocin: responsible for initiating the labor process and flow of breast milk

anterior pituitary

hypophysial vein

sella turcica

ADH: controls body's water balance

testosterone

TSH: stimulates thyroid to produce thyroid hormone

ACTH: stimulates adrenal glands to produce cortisone

prolactin: causes breast milk production

growth hormone: controls body's growth

FSH and LH: control estrogen, progesterone, and testosterone production

thyroid hormone

cortisone

estrogen

progesterone

▲ *Four of the pituitary hormones activate an organ to produce another related hormone. Some of this hormone in the blood will then feed back into the pituitary, thus regulating its production; some of it will also pass through the hypothalamus, stimulating neurosecretions that travel to the portal blood vessels and back into the pituitary to control the release of various other hormones.*

glands. FSH and LH in turn stimulate the production of two major sex hormones: estrogen and progesterone. These control menstruation in the female and stimulate the production of hormones and sperm in the male.

The hormone prolactin is one of two hormones of the anterior pituitary that seem to act on the body's tissues without stimulating other glands. Like gonadotropins, prolactin is concerned with reproduction. Also in common with gonadotropins, prolactin has a more complicated role in the female than in the male. Its role in the male is unclear, although excessive amounts can have ill effects. In the female, prolactin stimulates the breasts to produce milk. In large amounts, it also inhibits ovulation and the menstrual cycle. This explains why women who are breast-feeding are unlikely to conceive.

The anterior pituitary also produces growth hormone; its role is to promote normal growth. This is of most importance during childhood and adolescence, but the hormone continues to be of some importance in later life, since it determines the way that body tissues handle carbohydrates (see Growth).

What can go wrong
Since the pituitary plays such an important role, any malfunctions of the gland can be serious. However, such problems are quite unusual.

The pituitary may give rise to problems in three ways. Like any other gland, it may become either overactive or underactive; it may also be the site of a tumor. Since it lies in the base of the brain, tumors can cause problems by growing outward and pressing on important structures. For example, immediately above the sella is a structure called the optic chiasma, where the optic nerves that carry the information from the eyes cross over each other. Any slight pressure on the optic chiasma from an outward-growing pituitary tumor can lead to progressive loss of sight (see Tumors).

Tumors in the pituitary gland itself fall into two categories: those that produce excessive amounts of the various hormones, and those that do not. The most common type, prolactinomas, are very tiny;

however, they produce high levels of prolactin. In women, this overproduction will lead to amenorrhea (absence of periods), infertility, and sometimes galactorrhea (milk production from the breasts). In men, it can lead to impotence and sterility.

A second type of hormone-producing tumor leads to very high levels of growth hormone in the blood. If this starts before puberty, it leads to gigantism; this condition is rare, however. It is much more common for the condition to start in adulthood when the long bones of the arms and legs are no longer capable of growing. However, in such cases the affected person's hands and feet may grow thicker and his or her features may become gradually coarser

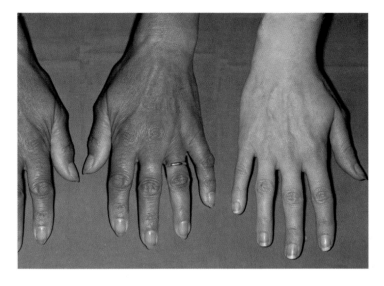

▲ *Darkening of the skin, shown in the two hands on the left, is a result of overactivity of the pituitary gland as it attempts to correct a deficiency of the adrenal glands.*

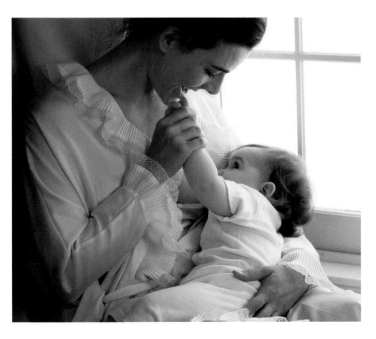

▲ *Two pituitary hormones are responsible for the production of breast milk: prolactin stimulates the breast to produce milk, and oxytocin triggers milk flow.*

as a result of new growth of facial bones. The nonbony parts of the body may also grow, leading to weight gain and thickening of the skin. When these problems occur, the condition is called acromegaly.

Another tumor makes ACTH, the hormone that stimulates the adrenals. This can lead to Cushing's syndrome, in which the adrenal glands produce too much cortisone. The condition results in obesity that is confined to the patient's abdomen and chest. The muscles in the arms and legs also become wasted; the skin becomes thin and bruises easily; and deep purple stretch marks may develop.

Tumors in or around the pituitary itself may affect the gland to the extent that it can no longer produce hormones. This can lead to hypopituitarism, which in adults may lead to a reduction in the gonadotropins secreted. Such a reduction usually results in a decline in sexual function in men, and amenorrhea in women; in both cases this can be distressing but it is not life-threatening.

If the thyroid gland or adrenal glands stop working properly, serious illness or even death can result. The main role of cortisone is to respond to stress, and it cannot do this if there is no ACTH to stimulate the adrenal glands when stress occurs. Doctors test the system by giving the patient an injection of insulin to lower the blood sugar; if the adrenal glands are working normally, the level of blood cortisone will be raised in response.

The posterior pituitary may also fail to produce hormones, although it is only the lack of ADH that causes difficulties. When ADH is absent, the body cannot retain water; this condition results in excessive thirst, and large amounts of urine are passed.

In children, an underactive pituitary can cause normal growth to be very slow, or to stop altogether. A lack of gonadotropins will also delay the onset of puberty. Tumors affecting the pituitary gland can occur in childhood, but are extremely rare. Children also occasionally suffer delayed growth as a result of a lack of growth hormone. In this condition, a tumor is not the cause.

Treatment

When problems with the pituitary cause disease, successful investigation depends on careful examination of the underlying hormonal problems. This can be exacting for both doctor and patient.

A small prolactinoma tumor may be treated by surgical removal. However, more often the resulting high prolactin levels are controlled with a drug called bromocriptine; this inhibits the release of prolactin. When there is an excess of growth hormone, surgery is more likely than it would be in a case of prolactinoma, because these tumors tend to be larger.

With Cushing's syndrome, tests must be performed to see if too much ACTH is produced by the pituitary, or if the problem is the adrenal glands. When the pituitary is at fault, the tiny pituitary tumor that is the cause may be removed by surgery.

For cortisone deficiency, cortisone tablets are given by mouth. Thyroid hormones, and sex hormones in women, are also given in this way using preparations similar to the contraceptive pill. In men, sex hormone replacement is best given by long-lasting injections or implants of testosterone (a male hormone). A deficiency of ADH is cured by giving the hormone in the form of a nasal spray.

Children who suffer from a lack of growth hormone can be treated successfully with injections of growth hormone.

See also: Adrenal glands; Glands; Hormones; Hypothalamus; Thyroid

Placebo effect

It may seem strange that patients can be cured of certain ailments by treatments that contain no active ingredient and exert no direct physical effect. However, this is exactly what happens sometimes with placebos.

A placebo is some form of medication, such as a pill or liquid, or a medical or surgical procedure that appears to be an orthodox medical aid but that has no active ingredient and no direct physical effect on the condition for which it is prescribed. This is not to say, however, that placebos have no place in medicine. They can often induce changes in a condition, alleviate various aches and pains, and make a sick person feel much better. They are also essential to medical research.

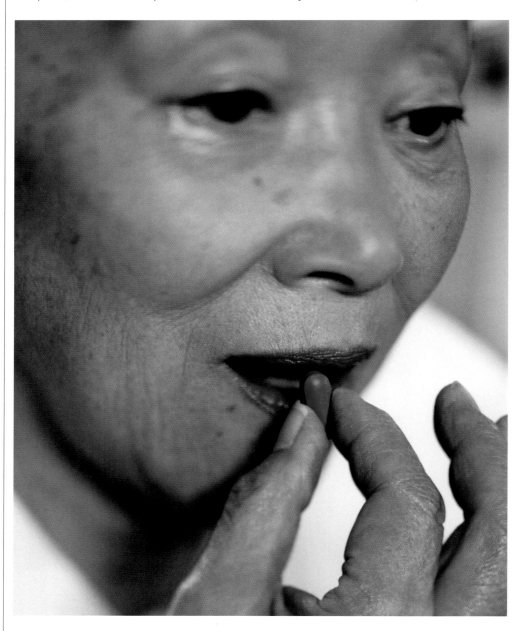

▲ *The central moral issue of placebo treatments is whether or not the ends justify the means. If the patient is cured, does it matter that he or she has been deceived?*

▶ *People do occasionally recover from disease without any scientific explanation. Some successes may be due to placebo treatments.*

An improvement that is effected by a placebo is not merely in the mind of the patient, although it may start that way. Physical changes do in fact result. Although these changes are not produced by the placebo directly, they occur as the result of changes in the patient's attitude, and his or her belief in what the placebo will do. The placebo effect is an excellent example of the power of the mind over the body.

Why placebos are used

Placebos are used in two medical situations. In the first, the patient is suffering from a disease or a condition in which the psychological control of the body state is at fault. In such a case, the condition is treated by causing the mind to induce a change in the functioning of the body.

For example, exhaustion that is due to anxiety can be cured by giving the patient a tonic that actually contains just a few vitamins. The patient does not know this, and the tonic causes him or her to believe that the fatigue will soon disappear. The placebo treatment therefore allows the patient to relax and release the anxiety that was causing the fatigue in the first place (see Anxiety; Fatigue).

In this way, a large number of diseases may be cured by a patient's simple expectation that an improvement will occur. Bodily changes then result, and it is these that actually cause the expected improvement to occur.

The second and a more important use of placebos is in medical research. Here the effectiveness of a new medication regimen or another treatment is compared with that of a similar-looking treatment that is in fact a placebo. This use is vital, because without it doctors could never be certain that any improvement shown as the result of taking a particular medication was not just due to an expectation on the part of the patient that the treatment would work.

When they are used

Placebos are not used indiscriminately. In normal medical practice their use is rare. Medicines, pills, and treatment regimens are nearly always genuine, because obviously the various drugs and treatments used in medicines are more powerful in their action than a pill that simply contains inactive ingredients.

In certain cases, however, the fewer medicines that enter a person's system, the better. If in such cases improvement can be brought about by psychological means, then a placebo treatment is preferable. There have even been cases of placebo surgery being carried out; such examples are, however, much more controversial than administering a placebo in the form of pills.

Clinical trials involving new medication with placebo control comparisons are never used on patients without their consent. If a person goes to a doctor for treatment, he or she will never be denied any real medication that is needed and given a placebo instead.

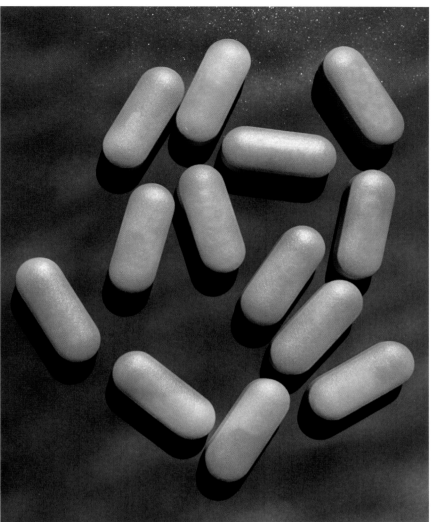

How they work

Very little is known about the way that placebos work, although there is clear evidence that a placebo can sometimes promote the release of endorphins that powerfully relieve pain.

Many of the cures effected by witch doctors, folk medicine, and faith healing involve the placebo principle. Indeed, faith healing claims openly that if a person believes that a given treatment will effect a cure, then a cure may sometimes be achieved.

Some people claim that a placebo can improve a patient's condition only if there is nothing physically wrong with the patient. However, this may not always be true, as some doctors have found to their surprise. Most doctors and researchers agree, therefore, that placebo treatment has an effect on the brain, which in turn gives out instructions that induce bodily activity. The bodily activity then helps to repair physical damage or malfunction in the patient.

There are some diseases that may be beyond the scope of the body's ability to cure itself. However, medical practice does encompass some apparently inexplicable cures. The possible powerful effect of placebos cannot be dismissed, however unlikely the circumstances may appear to be.

See also: **Faith healing; Medical research; Medicines; Mind; Mind-body therapy**

Placenta

Questions and Answers

Do twin babies share the same placenta?

When twins are identical it is because one fertilized egg has given rise to two babies. During their development they share a single placenta, but each baby grows in a separate sac.

Nonidentical twins grow from two separate eggs, so each baby has its own placenta.

My last baby was very small and I was told that this was because the placenta had not functioned well. What can I do next time to help my placenta function better?

Often there is no explanation for an unhealthy placenta, but as with all pregnancies it is important to eat well, get adequate rest, and attend prenatal clinics. Women with kidney disease, raised blood pressure, or heart disease are more likely to have small babies. If this applies to you, then you should talk to your doctor, who will be able to advise you about keeping as well as possible before you become pregnant. If you smoke, it is wise to stop before becoming pregnant, since smoking impairs placental function.

After I had my baby the doctor took a blood sample from the placenta. She said this was because my blood group is Rh-negative. Can you explain this?

Women whose blood group is Rh-negative can produce substances in their blood called Rh antibodies if the baby is Rh-positive. These antibodies cross the placenta, enter the baby's blood system, and can destroy some of the baby's blood cells, causing anemia. The blood in the large blood vessels of the placenta is the same as the baby's blood, and so it can be tested to check whether the baby is Rh-positive or Rh-negative.

During pregnancy the placenta provides the vital link between the mother and fetus. Both the feeding of the baby and the elimination of its waste products occur through this organ, which is expelled after the baby's birth.

ANATOMY OF THE PLACENTA

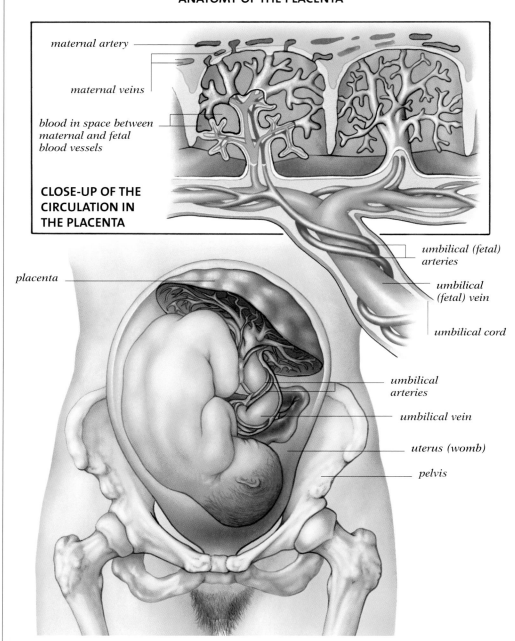

maternal artery

maternal veins

blood in space between maternal and fetal blood vessels

CLOSE-UP OF THE CIRCULATION IN THE PLACENTA

placenta

umbilical (fetal) arteries

umbilical (fetal) vein

umbilical cord

umbilical arteries

umbilical vein

uterus (womb)

pelvis

▲ *The placenta consists of maternal blood vessels in the uterine wall and fetal blood vessels, which arise from the umbilical cord. The exchange of food, oxygen, and waste products takes place in the spaces between the maternal and fetal blood vessels, which are not connected. Deoxygenated (blue) blood leaves the fetus along the umbilical arteries, and oxygenated (red) blood reaches the fetus via the umbilical vein.*

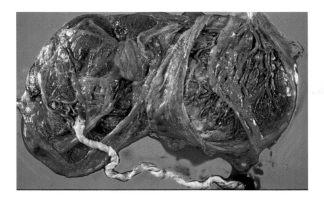

▲ *A placenta that supplied nourishment to twins. It was expelled shortly after the babies' birth.*

▶ *In the 10-week fetus the placenta is still immature and has a frilly, coral-like appearance.*

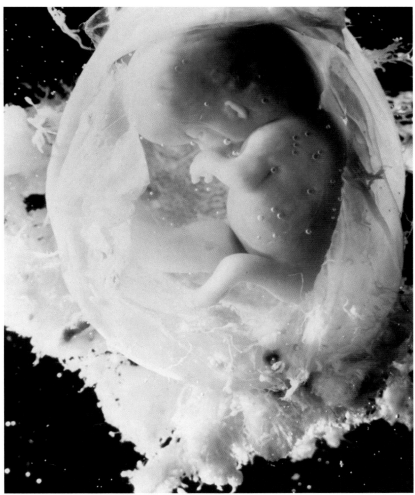

The placenta, or afterbirth, forms when a specialized part of the fertilized egg, the trophoblast, embeds in the wall of the mother's uterus. By the twelfth week of pregnancy, the placenta is an entirely separate organ. By the time the baby is born it will weigh a little over a pound (450 g) and will be dark red, spongy, and disk-shaped.

Two layers of cells keep the circulation of the fetal blood in the placenta separate from the mother's blood, but many substances can still pass from mother to baby.

The fetus receives all the food and oxygen it needs from its mother, and it is able to eliminate any waste products back into her circulation. This vital exchange function is carried out by the placenta, to which the fetus is attached by the umbilical cord. Oxygen, nutrients (simple carbohydrates, fats, and amino acids), and hormones pass from the mother to the fetus, and carbon dioxide, waste products, and hormones are transferred in the opposite direction.

The placenta also acts as a barrier to protect the fetus from potentially harmful substances, although many drugs can still cross the placenta and may damage the fetus. Some of the mother's antibodies also cross the placenta to protect the fetus.

Finally, the placenta produces hormones, some of which prevent the woman from releasing more eggs or menstruating while she is pregnant. These hormones also encourage breast development in preparation for breast-feeding, and the laying down of fat on the thighs, abdomen, and buttocks as a future energy store. Other placental hormones stimulate the growth of the uterus and probably prevent it from contracting before labor starts. There is also evidence to suggest that the amount of hormones released may be an important factor in determining when labor starts.

Monitoring the placenta

The absolute proof of a healthy placenta is the birth of a healthy baby. However, the efficiency of the placenta is often checked during pregnancy by measuring the amounts of hormones it releases into the mother's blood. Doctors assume that if the placenta is producing enough hormones, it is also working well in all other respects. If the hormone levels fall and it is suspected that the fetus is not receiving adequate nourishment, the baby may have to be delivered early.

Delivering the placenta

The placenta is normally delivered a few minutes after the baby's birth. The mother is given a shot of the hormone oxytocin, which causes the uterus to contract into a tight ball. The large maternal blood vessels to the placental site are then squeezed shut, and the placenta is sheared off the uterine wall. The obstetrician delivers the placenta through the vagina by pulling gently on the umbilical cord. He or she examines it afterward to ensure that it is complete.

Problems

Even a healthy placenta can cause occasional problems. In some rare cases it becomes partly or completely detached from the wall of the uterus before the baby is born, causing pain and bleeding. In such cases, urgent surgery is vital to save the lives of mother and baby.

In placenta previa, the placenta covers the neck of the womb completely, blocking the baby's passage through the birth canal. If this condition is present, the baby has to be delivered by cesarean section (see Cesarean Birth).

Sometimes a small piece of placenta does not come away in the normal manner at delivery and remains in the uterus. This can cause severe blood loss (secondary postpartum hemorrhage) several days after delivery. If an ultrasound shows a piece of retained placenta, an evacuation of the uterus must be performed.

See also: **Fetus; Pregnancy**

Plague

Questions and Answers

Is it possible for plague to erupt on the same scale as it did in the past?

Living conditions in many parts of the world have improved. We now know how the disease spreads, we have powerful rat poisons and insecticides, and antibiotics provide effective treatment. So although there may be small outbreaks of plague in poorer parts of the world, it is unlikely that a major outbreak on the scale of the great epidemics of the past could happen again. However, it is worth noting that in the aftermath of a nuclear war, the social chaos and collapse of public health services would be fertile ground for an epidemic.

Should I be vaccinated against plague if I go on a vacation in Asia?

Unless you spend your vacation in the most squalid conditions imaginable, you are unlikely to come into contact with the disease. The vaccine against plague provides protection for about six months and is intended only for people who, perhaps because of their occupation, have a high risk of exposure to the disease.

There are a large number of rats close to where I live. Is my family at risk from plague?

No, not unless you live in a part of the world where plague is a problem. However, rats do spread other diseases, and their presence is a sign of unsanitary conditions. You should make sure that action is taken to get rid of the rats.

Could plague bacteria ever be used in germ warfare between nations?

There is a form of plague known as pneumonic plague that might, in theory, be induced as a terrorist weapon, but plague is unsuitable for germ warfare and is unlikely to be effective in developed countries.

This devastating disease has been one of the scourges of humankind since time immemorial, and from time to time it still erupts in many parts of the world, in places where hygiene and living conditions are poor.

Plague is one of the most deadly infectious diseases known to humankind. At different times in history it has wreaked havoc with the populations of entire continents. The name "plague" was once used for any disease that caused a large number of deaths, but it is now used only for the disease caused by the bacterium *Yersinia pestis*.

History

There have been three major epidemic cycles, each one lasting many years and taking the lives of an enormous number of people. The first was in the sixth century; it lasted more than 50 years and spread over the whole Roman world. The second, in the 14th century, was known as the "black death" and devastated the population of Europe. It is estimated that a quarter of all the people on the continent died during this epidemic.

The Great Plague of London in 1664–1665 was not part of a major cycle, but it was deadly in its own right. In one year, 70,000 of London's population of 460,000 were killed by the disease.

The most recent epidemic cycle began in 1855 in China. It spread all over the world in an epidemic that lasted over 60 years. The recorded number of deaths from the plague between 1896 and 1917 was more than 10 million.

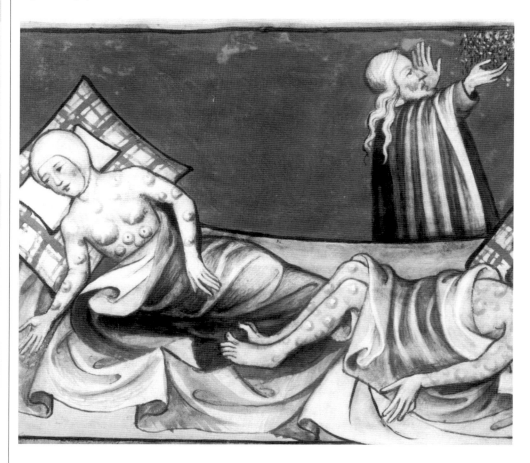

▲ *This painting from the Toggenberg bible shows people in the 15th century covered in abscesses; they are suffering from the bubonic plague.*

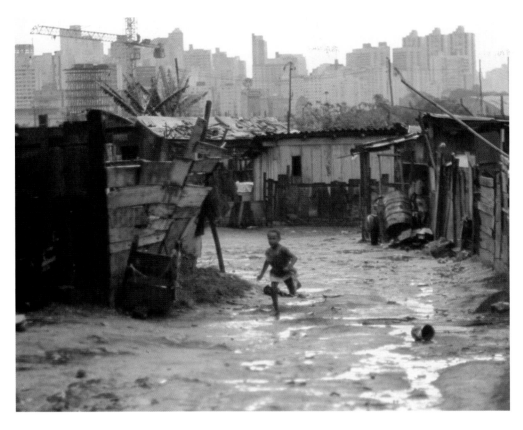

nodes usually appear in the groin and contain pus. They are called buboes, and the disease is therefore sometimes called bubonic plague. The internal bleeding often produces large dark bruises under the skin; for that reason, plague used to be called the "black death" (see Bruises).

Plague causes a severe type of pneumonia, and the disease spreads rapidly from one person to another through the coughing and sneezing that occur (see Pneumonia). This pneumonic plague is highly contagious, and without treatment it is rapidly fatal. The famous nursery rhyme "ring-around-a-rosy" is actually about plague: the roses refer to the petechiae (red spots) that appear over the buboes; the phrase "pocket full of posies" refers to the flowers that were carried to mask the smell; and the phrase "Atishoo! Atishoo! We all fall down!" refers to the violent sneezing—and ultimate death.

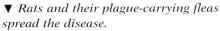

▲ *Unsanitary conditions make an ideal breeding ground for plague.*

▼ *Rats and their plague-carrying fleas spread the disease.*

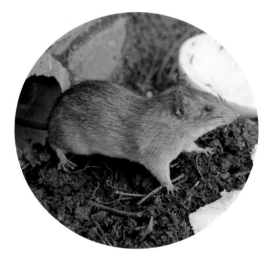

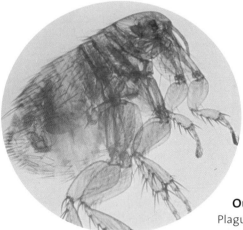

Treatment

With prompt treatment, plague can be completely cured. The most effective antibiotics available are aminoglycosides, tetracyclines, and sulfonamides, which are given in large doses. The buboes must be lanced to allow the pus to drain (see Pus).

In an epidemic, isolation of all cases of plague, rat extermination measures, vaccination, and widespread spraying to kill the fleas that carry the disease are needed (see Parasites). The insecticide must be chosen with great care; in the past, excessive use of DDT enhanced the fleas' resistance to this substance.

Outlook

Plague is still found in wild rodents everywhere except Australia; in parts of Asia, Africa, and South America people still contract the disease. There is even the occasional case in the United States.

Plague is most commonly associated with squalid living conditions in places heavily infested with rats and fleas. Hunters and trappers are also occasionally at risk, as are longshoremen and ship handlers.

Causes

The bacterium *Yersinia pestis* (formerly *Pasteurella pestis*) is carried by fleas that normally live on the bodies of wild rodents that have little or no contact with people. The disease is transmitted by flea bites. Sometimes the disease is transmitted to rats, which have much closer access to people. When the rats die, their fleas have to find new hosts and transfer to humans, who become infected.

Symptoms

Once the bacteria enter the body, they cause a sudden high fever, with collapse, internal bleeding, swollen lymph nodes, abscesses, and pneumonia (see Abscess; Lymphatic System). The swollen lymph

As living conditions around the world slowly improve, the number of plague victims continues to fall. But because the disease is established in wild rodents it is unlikely to disappear completely.

See also: Antibiotics; Bacteria; Hygiene; Immunization; Public Health; Tetracyclines; Vaccinations

Plaque

If people look at their teeth in a mirror, they may notice a yellowish-white deposit. This is plaque, one of the primary causes of tooth decay and gum disease. With good dental care its harmful effects can be minimized.

Questions and Answers

How can I tell if I have plaque?

Plaque shows up as a soft, whitish-yellow material, either near to the gum's edge or on areas where teeth overlap. Bleeding gums are also a sign that plaque is present.

To find out whether your teeth have plaque, you can use a disclosing agent (a colored tablet that you chew). This stains plaque pink, but does not affect the teeth themselves. Plaque deposits can then be removed most effectively by a dental hygienist.

Does plaque cause bad breath?

There are several causes of bad breath (halitosis). The most common cause is poor teeth and gums, which may develop because of plaque deposits. Plaque can cause halitosis, as can gum breakdown, caused by the bacteria in plaque. Dental care may eliminate bad breath, but people with halitosis should also check with a dental hygienist.

Is a soft or a hard toothbrush better for plaque removal?

Neither. A soft brush is seldom effective enough to remove plaque, and a hard brush may damage teeth and gums. A rotary-action electric toothbrush with a medium bristle will probably be the most suitable and effective.

Can eating certain foods prevent plaque formation?

There is no way to prevent plaque formation entirely. However, foods containing a fibrous material have a cleansing effect, and are preferable to soft foods that stick between teeth. The best way to prevent plaque accumulation is to take good care of your teeth, and to restrict your intake of sugar. This will limit acid production in plaque and minimize tooth decay.

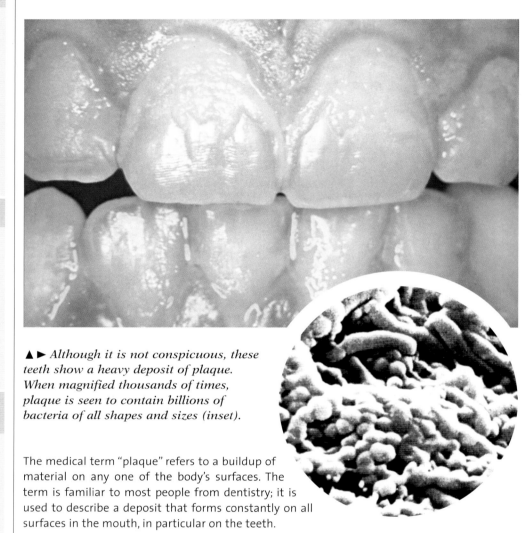

▲ ▶ *Although it is not conspicuous, these teeth show a heavy deposit of plaque. When magnified thousands of times, plaque is seen to contain billions of bacteria of all shapes and sizes (inset).*

The medical term "plaque" refers to a buildup of material on any one of the body's surfaces. The term is familiar to most people from dentistry; it is used to describe a deposit that forms constantly on all surfaces in the mouth, in particular on the teeth.

Plaque is a whitish-yellow sticky material that may be invisible to the naked eye. However, it becomes highly visible once it has accumulated. Because it spreads and clings to teeth, it can cause a great deal of damage to teeth and gums. Correct and regular brushing, along with use of dental floss, will prevent plaque and lessen the chances of tooth decay and gum disease.

What is plaque?

Plaque is made up of bacteria and their by-products, together with the constituents of saliva. The bacteria in plaque are of many types, and are classified according to their shape: spherical (cocci), rods (bacilli), filaments, and spirals (see Bacteria). Bacteria are not visible to the naked eye, but vast numbers may be present; it has been estimated that the plaque between any two teeth contains perhaps two billion bacteria.

Plaque is formed by bacteria that are enclosed in a sticky material composed of proteins. This sticky material is derived from the saliva, together with polysaccharides and glycoproteins, which are derived from the plaque bacteria. Food debris is also present, although not in very significant amounts.

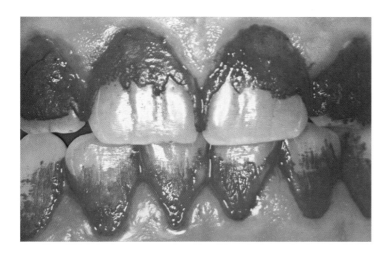

▲ *A disclosing agent (a tablet that is chewed) will stain the teeth in places where plaque is present.*

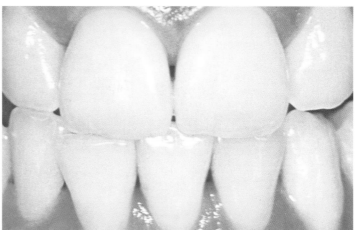

▲ *Only when the deposits of plaque have been removed will the teeth be truly clean.*

Plaque bacteria will thrive especially when other organisms, such as yeasts and viruses, are present in the mouth.

Sometimes plaque may exist only as a thin, invisible film. However, if it is allowed to build up, it may become thicker. Plaque that has accumulated over a long period may eventually calcify, and it is then known as calculus or tartar. This, unlike plaque, is a hard deposit.

How plaque is formed

The bacteria involved in plaque formation are present in the mouth from birth. Once teeth begin to emerge, they become coated with a glycoprotein layer, which is derived from the saliva. This forms a thin skin—or pellicle—over the teeth. Subsequently, bacteria from the saliva adhere to the pellicle and multiply, forming colonies. The first bacteria to do this are round and rod-shaped types; these bacteria then derive oxygen from the saliva.

Later, organisms that do not require oxygen begin to multiply deep within the plaque; these organisms are called anaerobes. As the plaque layer thickens, spiral bacteria and filamentous bacteria also begin to multiply, and these constitute a significant part of the plaque flora. Over a period of time, this layer of plaque thickens to the stage where it is clearly visible as a surface deposit on the teeth.

Effects of plaque

The bacteria of plaque are responsible for both tooth decay and periodontal disease—that is, disease of the gums and tissues that hold the teeth in position.

The progressive breakdown and crumbling of the enamel and dentine of a tooth, leading to the formation of a cavity within the tooth, is known medically as dental caries. Enamel and dentine are both hard tissues, and are very strong mechanically. However, it is still possible for them to be dissolved by chemicals such as acids.

The bacteria within plaque produce significant amounts of acid when given a source of sucrose. The main source of sucrose in the mouth comes from the breakdown of carbohydrates; sucrose is also the main constituent of sugar.

Within only a few minutes after a person eats candy or food that contains sugar, the acidity adjacent to the tooth surfaces rises to a critical level and the tooth enamel starts to dissolve. Even when the person stops eating, this process may continue for up to half an hour.

Tooth decay

Tooth decay, therefore, depends on a number of factors: plaque; the amount of sugar in a person's diet; and the amount of resistance that a person's tooth enamel has to decay. If plaque could be eliminated, tooth decay could also be prevented. However, it is possible only to reduce, rather than to entirely remove, all traces of plaque. For this reason, the most effective methods currently available for preventing tooth decay include controlling the amount of sugar a person eats, protecting tooth enamel with the use of fluoride, either by fluoridation of water or in a toothpaste, and sealing the crevices within the teeth's surfaces in which plaque would otherwise be likely to form.

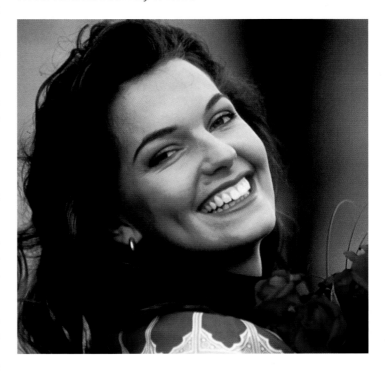

▲ *If you take care of your teeth with regular and careful brushing, and reduce your sugar intake, you will lessen the chances of tooth decay and gum disease.*

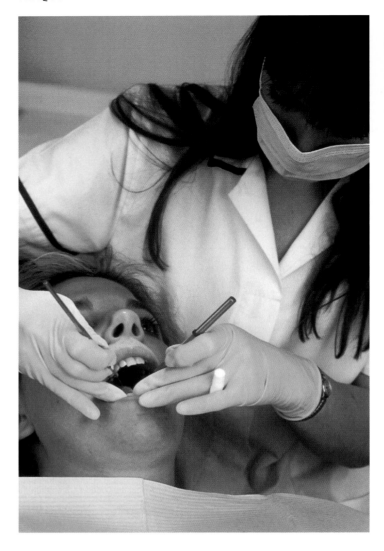

▲ *The only way to prevent tooth decay and gum disease is by correct and regular brushing. While this dental hygienist will clean the teeth properly, her main task will be to show patients how to do this themselves.*

In the case of chronic periodontal disease, the process by which plaque damages the gum and other structures is—as with tooth decay—caused by the products of bacterial metabolism. However, with gum disease the process is different in that the damaging factor is not acid, but the production of toxic organic chemicals by the plaque bacteria.

Chronic periodontal disease is present to some degree in most people. The condition involves a slow, progressive destruction of the many tissues that hold the teeth in position, leading eventually to tooth loss. Periodontal disease is so widespread that people often accept tooth loss as an inevitable result of aging. However, if effective measures are taken to remove plaque, tooth loss can be prevented.

How to avoid plaque

At present, it is impossible to avoid the formation of plaque, because the bacteria involved are the normal inhabitants of the mouth. Immunization techniques and the long-term use of antibiotics have both been tried, but neither method is effective. In the former there

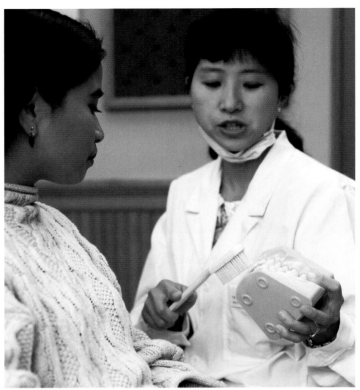

▲ *The best way to prevent plaque is to teach children how to brush and the importance of brushing from an early age.*

are too many types of bacteria to counteract, and in the latter the bacteria would eventually build up resistance to the antibiotic used. Antiseptics have also been tried, but long-term use causes tooth discoloration and, over time, resistance may also occur.

Therefore, the measures to be taken center on preventive methods (see Preventive Medicine). Teeth should be brushed at least once a day, but thorough brushing is more important than the number of times teeth are brushed. The type of brush that should be used is flat-headed, with medium bristles, and a short, straight handle, since this can reach into awkward corners of the mouth. Teeth should be brushed for about three minutes, from the gum downward or upward, since each area must be brushed several times to remove the plaque, which is very sticky. An electric toothbrush will make plaque removal far less laborious; but water irrigation devices will not completely remove all the plaque, because plaque clings too strongly to the teeth.

Those areas that are not accessible to the toothbrush, such as between the teeth, should be cleaned by using dental floss. The waxed and unwaxed varieties are equally effective, but the waxed kind may feel smoother, particularly if the teeth are close together.

If people restrict the amount of sugar in their diet, they will limit acid production by plaque and so will help minimize tooth decay. When a low-sugar diet is combined with other measures against tooth decay, it is possible for the teeth to remain cavity-free. Chronic periodontal disease can also be limited by this preventive action.

See also: **Dental care; Gums and gum diseases; Halitosis; Pyorrhea and gingivitis; Saliva; Teeth and teething**

Plasma

Questions and Answers

Can a blood donor give just plasma without the other parts of the blood?

When people give blood, whole blood is normally taken, but it may then be separated into its component parts so that more patients benefit. In exceptional circumstances, blood can be taken with a cell-separating machine so that just the plasma is removed. For example, this technique might be used when antibodies to a disease such as hepatitis are needed to protect people who have been exposed to the virus.

Can someone run out of plasma or get sick by having too little?

Keeping an adequate amount of plasma in the circulation is such a central part of the body's activities that when this function breaks down, the whole body suffers. It is thus a matter of urgency when major bleeding or dehydration causes a loss of circulatory fluid. In emergency situations, doctors can replace much of the lost volume with saline rather than plasma, limiting the need for transfusions.

When my brother was in the hospital he was connected to a machine that took the blood from his body and then put it back again. Why was this done?

It is possible to take blood from the body, separate the cells from the plasma, and then return the cells in a citric-saline or similar solution—a process called plasmapheresis. The technique is used when the plasma contains a substance that is harmful to the patient. For example, the plasma may contain a harmful antibody, or an excessive amount of a certain protein that makes the blood thick and sticky so that it doesn't flow along the blood vessels properly.

Plasma is the fluid in which the red and white blood cells are suspended. It also contains many dissolved substances, including proteins and minerals, that are essential to life.

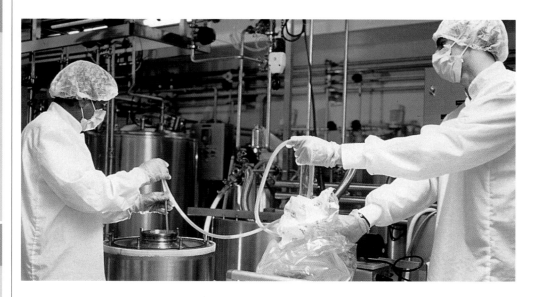

▲ *Blood bank technicians withdraw plasma from a machine that separates raw blood into its components. It is then frozen and stored until it is needed for transfusion.*

Plasma, the fluid component of blood, transports the red and white blood cells around the body. It consists mainly of water, but also contains water-soluble substances (see Blood). Some of these substances are important to the body. They include body fuels such as glucose and basic fats; minerals such as iron, which is essential for the formation of the oxygen-carrying pigment hemoglobin; and other vital compounds, such as thyroid hormone. Others, such as carbon dioxide, are waste products that need to be expelled from the body.

Since plasma is a liquid, it can diffuse through the walls of the capillaries by osmosis, and mix with the extracellular fluid that bathes the surface of all the body's cells (see Capillaries). As a result, soluble substances can be carried from cell to cell.

Plasma proteins

Protein is the most abundant of the soluble substances in the plasma: each quart (liter) of plasma contains about $2\frac{1}{2}$ ounces (75 g) of protein. There are two main types: albumin and globulin.

Albumin, which is manufactured in the liver, is a source of food for the tissues and also provides the osmotic pressure that keeps the plasma inside the blood vessels and stops it from flooding out into the body tissues. Albumin can be thought of as a circulating liquid sponge that keeps necessary water in the bloodstream and so stops the whole body from degenerating into a damp mass of tissue. Of the globulins, possibly the most important are those that act as antibodies against infection (see Immune System). Others are active in the formation of blood clots.

Plasma transfusions

Blood from donors is often separated into its two main components, cells and plasma. Plasma transfusions may be given when people have lost a large amount of blood and lack the circulatory fluid to enable their heart to beat effectively, to counteract severe bleeding, and to boost immune function.

See also: Blood donor; Blood transfusion; Fats; Glucose; Hormones; Minerals

Plastic and reconstructive surgery

Surgery that is performed to improve the shape of a nose or remove wrinkles is only a minor part of an important branch of medicine; its major concern is with the repair or reconstruction of damaged or deformed tissues.

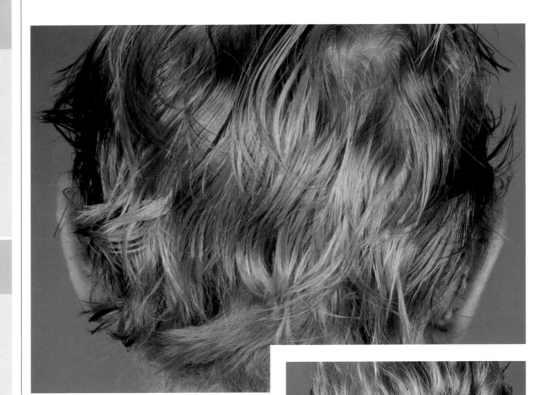

▲ ▶ *Protruding ears (right) can cause people great embarrassment, but they can be treated by plastic surgery (above).*

The term "plastic surgery" simply means any surgery that changes the shape of the body, but it is now also used to mean surgery in which tissues are moved from one part of the body to another. Because skin is one of the tissues in the body that can be moved relatively easily from one place to another, plastic surgery has tended to become synonymous with skin grafting, but many other techniques are used by the plastic surgeon.

Conditions requiring treatment

Plastic surgery deals with a wide range of conditions, including congenital abnormalities (conditions that people are born with), injuries such as burns and crushed hands, and disfigurements and scars resulting from diseases such as cancer of the skin or of the lining of the mouth (see Cancer).

Among the congenital abnormalities that a plastic surgeon may treat are cleft lip and palate, conditions that can occur together. Correction of these defects not only makes a truly remarkable

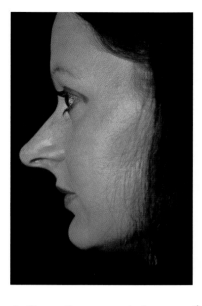

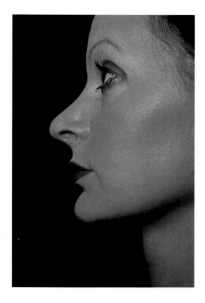

▲ *Cosmetic surgery to improve the shape of the nose can achieve a dramatic change in the appearance of the patient, as shown in the photographs above, taken before and after surgery. Surgery is done under general anesthesia and the patient will usually have to spend several days in the hospital before being discharged.*

improvement in a person's appearance, but also is necessary for the normal development of speech and the proper growth of teeth. A cleft lip is usually corrected when a baby is about three months old, although some surgeons prefer to make the repair when the infant is much younger. The palate is repaired at about nine months to one year, which is before the time when speech development begins (see Cleft Palate).

Children who have birthmarks are often referred to plastic surgeons. Many birthmarks, such as the strawberry nevus, do not normally require any surgery, because they often disappear as the child grows older. However, surgery may be needed if complications develop, such as bleeding from the birthmark or obstruction of the baby's eyesight (see Birthmarks).

There are a number of other congenital deformities that may need plastic surgery, although none of them is particularly common. A baby may have extra fingers or toes (polydactyly), fingers that are joined together (syndactyly), or extra tags of skin around the earlobes (accessory auricle). Occasionally, the penis is slightly abnormal, with the opening on the underside instead of at the tip (hypospadias). Because none of these conditions is very dangerous, there is no real urgency to correct them and surgery is usually left until the child is older. At this age the operation and the administration of anesthesia are less demanding (see Anesthetics).

REMOVING BAGS FROM UNDER THE EYES

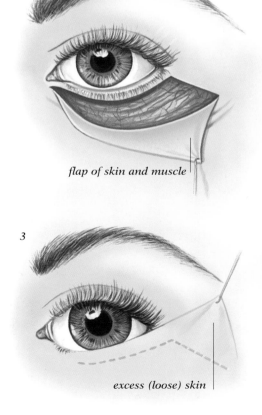

1 flap of skin and muscle

2 excess fat

3 excess (loose) skin

4 stitches

◄ *This operation is usually performed under local anesthesia. The surgeon makes an incision under the patient's lower eyelid to pull down a flap of skin and muscle (1); in some cases, it is also necessary to remove excess fat from beneath the skin (2). The surgeon then pulls the skin and muscle from the flap upward at the outer corner of the patient's eye and removes the excess tissue by making a triangular cut (3). The incisions are closed with small stitches (4), which are usually removed 48 to 72 hours after the surgery. Under normal circumstances, the healed tissue will leave tiny scars that will be barely visible when they are covered with a light layer of makeup. Although this type of surgery is most frequently carried out to conceal the effects of aging, it may also be performed on young people to remove excess fat that is an inherited facial characteristic.*

My daughter has spina bifida. Can plastic surgery be of any help?

The handicap resulting from spina bifida is caused by the nerves in the spinal cord being permanently damaged by the congenital defect in the back. Paralysis of the legs and other factors, such as loss of feeling and bladder weakness, are a result of this damage. Although surgery can be performed to cover any exposed nervous system tissue in the lower back, it can only alleviate the complications and can never cure the basic problem.

When I was young I had several tattoos done. I am now married and in a responsible job and am self-conscious about these tattoos. Can they be removed by plastic surgery or by other means?

You may find a plastic surgeon who is sympathetic to your request if the tattoos are interfering with your working relationships or marriage. Laser treatment is found to be most effective for removal of tattoos. Lasers penetrate the outer layer of skin and break up the pigment. It is a costly and painful process and several treatments will be required. Tattoos cannot be eliminated completely by laser treatment; a faint trace of the tattoo will remain. Dermabrasion is another method; the tattoo is sprayed with a solution to freeze the skin; the tattoo is then sanded with a rotary instrument. Some bleeding may occur, and a dressing will be applied.

Is the risk of cancer higher in women who have breast implants?

Breast implants have not been shown to cause cancer. However, in a patient who has had a mastectomy (removal of the breast) for cancer, the use of an implant to rebuild the absent breast might mask a recurrence of the disease. Many surgeons therefore prefer to wait several years after a mastectomy—until the chances of a recurrent cancer are minimal—before they will consider breast reconstruction.

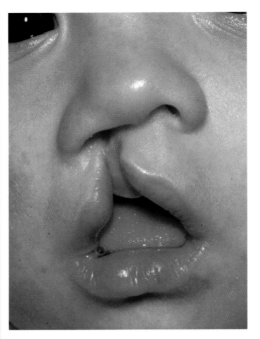

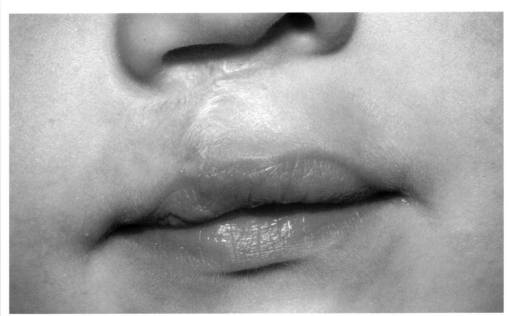

Severe burns may require the attention of the plastic surgeon both at the time of the injury and at a later date to improve the look of scars that may develop. If the burns are of partial thickness (the deeper layers of skin are not damaged) they will heal naturally. Areas where the burns are of full thickness, when even the deepest layers in the skin have been damaged, will require skin grafts. Once the burned area is covered with skin it becomes much less painful.

Replantation, sewing back a part of the body that has been accidentally amputated, is a beneficial advance, but there are many technical difficulties. Only certain amputation

◄ ▼ *Modern surgical techniques enable plastic surgeons to correct congenital deformities such as cleft lip (left), so that the mouth and nose will develop normally after surgery (below).*

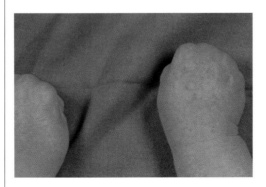

▲ *In complete syndactyly, a congenital abnormality of the hand, the baby's fingers are completely fused.*

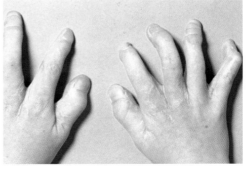

▲ *At first glance the condition would appear hopeless, but plastic surgery produces excellent results.*

FACE-AND-NECK LIFT (RHYTIDECTOMY)

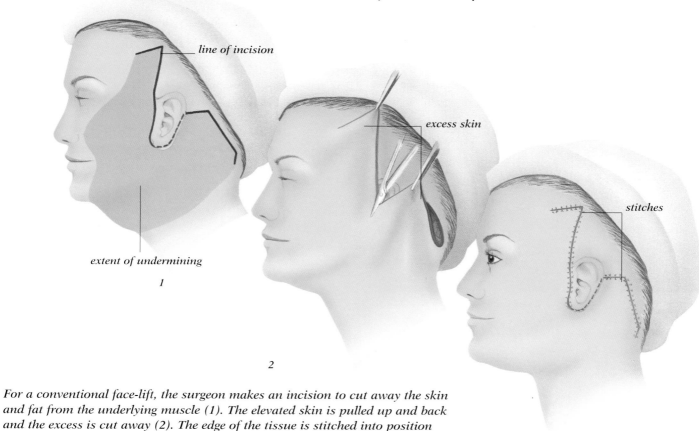

line of incision

excess skin

stitches

extent of undermining

1

2

3

For a conventional face-lift, the surgeon makes an incision to cut away the skin and fat from the underlying muscle (1). The elevated skin is pulled up and back and the excess is cut away (2). The edge of the tissue is stitched into position (3). In most cases, the scar tissue will soon be hidden by the growth of new hair.

injuries, such as the loss of a whole thumb, hand, or arm, may be suitable for replantation (see Hand). During surgery, the blood vessels are rejoined with the aid of an operating microscope (microvascular surgery). Repairs are also made to the bones, tendons, arteries, nerves, veins, and skin. However, it is unusual for the patient to regain completely normal sensation in the limb or digit after such severe injury (see Nervous System).

Severe lacerations to the face are often referred to a plastic surgeon. Such injuries most commonly result when a person who is not wearing a seat belt is thrown through the windshield of a car (see Lacerations).

When skin growths or lumps have been surgically removed, plastic surgery may be needed to repair defects in the skin and underlying tissue.

Cosmetic surgery

Cosmetic surgery can improve the features of the face, such as by straightening the nose or tightening sagging tissues under the chin or eyelids. Surgery is usually done under general anesthesia, and the patient usually spends a day or two in the hospital.

Breasts may be increased in size by inserting artificial implants, or prostheses, deep into the breast tissue (see Breasts). The prostheses are plastic bags filled with saline or silicone, and they are designed to mimic the texture and shape of a real breast (see Prostheses). Sensation in the nipple may be temporarily changed by surgery, but breast-feeding is still possible, since the breast tissue is not damaged. Surgery to reduce the size of the breasts involves

cutting through the breast tissue and, as a result, breast-feeding is not possible (see Breast-Feeding).

Surgery can also be carried out to reduce the amount of fat and loose skin on the stomach, thighs, and buttocks (see Liposuction). The plastic surgeon tries to make the long scars that result as unobtrusive as possible—for example, by putting them in the bikini area if this is feasible. Before undergoing cosmetic surgery, the patient should discuss it with the family doctor. While cosmetic surgeons can make considerable improvements to a person's appearance, they cannot perform miracles, so it is best for the person to find out what will be involved and whether the reasons for wanting the change justify the surgery.

Skin grafts

Skin grafting is a common technique used by plastic surgeons to cover raw areas, such as those that result from severe burns. Every effort is made to match the skin that is being grafted with that in the area surrounding the wound in color, texture, and hairiness.

Partial-thickness or split-skin grafts are commonly taken from the inside or back of the thighs, or from the buttocks or inner upper arms. This type of graft may involve only the epidermis (the outer layer of skin), but usually some of the dermis (the inner layer) is also included. Because the whole layer of skin is not removed, the skin can regrow over the area from which the graft is taken. It does this by spreading out from the epithelial cells that are left behind in hair follicles and sweat glands (see Perspiration). The area will normally heal like a superficial graze, with little scarring.

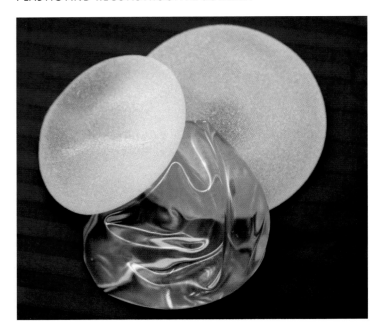

▲ *The different types of breast implants include one filled with a soft fluidlike silicone gel, one with a solid jellylike silicone gel, and one with a saline (salt and water) solution. All these implants are surrounded by a firm, elastic silicone shell.*

In some cases the whole layer of skin needs to be grafted, in what is called a full-thickness graft. Here the skin around the area from which the graft is taken must be sewn together, because no epithelial cells are left behind.

Grafts in which skin is completely removed from the donor area are called free skin grafts. Often, however, a skin flap, or pedicle, has to be used to fill a defect. A flap consists of skin and fat, or skin, fat, and muscle. Unlike a free skin graft, however, it must have an adequate blood supply at all times during the transfer to keep it alive.

Grafting techniques

If a split-skin graft is used, the skin is removed from one part of the body and laid over the defect that needs to be closed. The raw area is first carefully prepared to make certain that it is clean and free from infection (see Infection and Infectious Diseases). This preparation may be done over a period of days or weeks in the patient's hospital room, or it may be done under anesthesia in the operating room, depending on the nature of the original defect. For example, an ulcer on the leg due to disease of the veins may be badly infected and may need some days or weeks of treatment before grafting is attempted, whereas a defect left by surgery could be grafted right away. Infection under a graft often results in complete failure of the graft to take.

When the area to be grafted has been prepared, the skin graft is taken. This is done with an instrument called a dermatome. The dermatome may be one of two types: a handheld instrument that is like a large razor blade, with an adjustable stop to vary the thickness of the graft; or an electric knife that runs over the skin like an electric plane. Both types allow the surgeon to take an extremely fine layer of skin containing live cells. If too thick a graft is taken, the skin cannot grow back and the patient is left with a defect at this site.

A split-skin graft consists of an extremely fine layer of skin, so fine that it is transparent. It must be handled very carefully to avoid damage and is usually spread out onto a layer of Vaseline gauze. It sticks to the gauze, which makes it easier to cut it to the right size to graft the defect. The skin is then laid on to the raw surface and either stitched into position or held in position by a special dressing. The donor area is covered with Vaseline gauze and a pressure dressing (see Dressings and Bandages).

The dressings on both the donor and the recipient sites are usually left in position for about seven to 10 days. If the dressing over the graft is removed too early, there may be some danger of dislodging the graft. However, after a week it is usually obvious whether the graft has taken. If it has, it appears as a healthy pink area; if it hasn't, there is usually an accumulation of fluid under the graft, which is floating around and not stuck to the defect.

When a skin flap or pedicle is used to fill a defect, most of the flap of tissue is raised, but it is left attached at one edge of the donor area. It will remain attached in this way even after the flap has been stitched to the raw area so that the flap has an uninterrupted blood flow. The flap will not be completely detached until it has established its own blood supply.

One of the main problems in grafting large areas, especially after burns, is that a patient may not have enough unaffected skin from which to take grafts. This problem can now be helped by using cellular wound dressings, which are a temporary covering to help prevent infection and fluid loss until autografting can be done. In some ways, wound dressings replace two layers of skin. The top layer of a wound dressing simulates the epidermis; after a while, it peels away or skin grafts replace it. The bottom layer of the dressing is a type of matrix that supports cells and promotes the growth of new skin. Nerve fibers and blood vessels from healthy tissue around the burn enter this matrix and combine with the cells of the wound dressing. Eventually, the matrix disappears as a new dermis forms. One such new generation of cellular wound dressing is Transcyte, which consists of human cells grown onto nylon mesh, and combined with a synthetic epidermal layer. Wound dressings reduce time in the hospital, relieve pain, and promote healing.

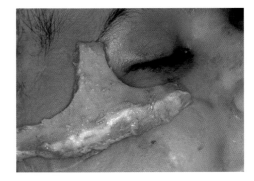
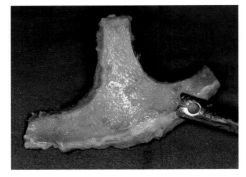

▲ *Pieces of bone can be grafted onto an area where there is a deficiency—for example, when an injury has left a depression in the cheekbone. This bone graft was taken from the patient's pelvis.*

Types of plastic surgery
Cosmetic surgery
Face-lift
Rhinoplasty (changing the shape of the nose)
Breast augmentation or reduction
Apronectomy (removing the apron of skin hanging from the abdomen in obese people who have lost weight)
Congenital abnormalities
Cleft lip and cleft palate
Abnormalities of the fingers
Skin grafting
Used to treat burns, after surgery to remove skin tumors, after severe trauma
Other types of grafting (muscle, bone, tendon)
Used to treat deformity or injury

Bone grafting

Pieces of bone can also be grafted into an area where there is a deficiency of bone—for example, if an injury has left a depression in the cheekbone or skull. Bone grafts are usually taken from the pelvis or ribs, and this procedure does not cause any permanent disability. Similarly, a graft of cartilage may be taken from the ear and used in the patient's nose.

Although it is preferable to use bone material from the patient's own body in an operation, it is sometimes necessary to take the material from a donor. However, donor grafts are not as readily accepted by the body, so there are often difficulties associated with their use (see Donors). To minimize these difficulties, the bone must be specially treated before it is grafted, but even then it may be rejected by the surrounding body tissues. Metals and plastics used in place of bone may cause similar problems.

Scars and scarring

All surgical incisions leave a scar, and plastic surgery is no exception. However, the plastic surgeon, through his or her training in dealing with delicate body tissue and knowledge of healing wounds, will try to achieve the best possible scar under the circumstances (see Healing). He or she may also plan the incisions in such a way that the final scars will be disguised by wrinkles or natural folds in the skin of the patient.

The extent of scarring following plastic surgery depends on several factors, including the patient's tendency to form thickened (or hypertrophic) scars and whether or not any infection develops in the wound after surgery (see Wounds). It also depends on the type of surgery that is performed. For example, surgery to make the breasts larger usually leaves just two small scars in the crease under the breasts; but surgery to make the breasts smaller requires more extensive incisions and is therefore likely to produce more extensive scarring, both under the breasts and around the nipples.

The plastic surgeon can also deal with scars that are already present. He or she can do this in a number of different ways. The scar can be cut out (excised) and the skin on each side simply sewn together again. The surgeon will do his or her best to prevent the conditions that may have caused the original scar (such as infection, bleeding into the wound, or too much tension on the stitches) from occurring again, and thus producing a similar scar. He or she may insert several stitches deep into the skin so that tension is taken off the skin edges. This means that the surface stitches can probably be taken out two or three days after surgery, and there is then less likelihood that the stitches will leave the familiar puncture marks along each side of the wound.

If the gap left by the excision of the scar is too wide to suture, the surgeon can do one of two things. First, he or she can cut under the skin on each side, making it possible to slide the skin over the muscles underneath. Second, he or she can put a skin graft over the defect. If a split-skin graft is used, the cosmetic result is never as good as if a full-thickness graft is used. Unless a full-thickness graft is very small, it will involve complicated surgery to move the tissue while retaining its blood supply.

Problems

There are two main difficulties that can cause poor results in plastic surgery: infection and poor blood supply. The former can be counteracted by meticulous attention to detail in performing an operation, together with the use of antibiotics in special cases (see Antibiotics). The problem of blood supply can be overcome only by a sound knowledge of the anatomy of the blood supply system and the various structures involved (see Circulatory System), as well as avoidance of tension on the body tissues.

Outlook

Plastic surgery can be very successful—for example, in the treatment of congenital deformities such as polydactyly and syndactyly. A baby whose fingers or toes are completely joined at birth can initially cause his or her parents considerable concern, but the condition can be treated by plastic surgery, usually with remarkable results.

Good results can also be produced in the treatment of facial scars and the augmentation or reduction of breast tissue.

When skin or muscle has to be moved from one part of the body to another, the patient may have to undergo surgery on a number of occasions and spend many months in the hospital.

It should also be mentioned that there is virtually no possibility of completely removing a scar by plastic surgery. The scar can be made less prominent and possibly cleverly hidden in a natural crease in the skin, but the idea that a plastic surgeon can somehow make scars invisible is a myth.

See also: **Burns; Congenital disorders; Cosmetic surgery; Grafting; Mastectomy; Microsurgery; Scars; Skin and skin diseases; Surgery; Sutures**

Pleurisy

Questions and Answers

Is pleurisy always painful?

Pleurisy usually causes pain, which is made worse by deep breathing, since the two inflamed layers of the pleura rub against each other. If the two layers of the pleura are separated, as happens in a pleural effusion, the pain may stop.

Can pleurisy cause permanent damage to the lungs or the pleura?

Yes. This happens particularly in tuberculosis and other bacterial infections in which pleural infection tends to leave thick scars on the surface of the pleura. Sometimes the scarring becomes even thicker as a result of infiltration by calcium, and in very rare cases this process can lead to the lungs' becoming encased in a hard bony cage.

How soon after having pleurisy can a normal life be resumed?

This will depend on the original cause of the pleurisy, and how fit you were to begin with. After an attack of pleurisy due to a viral infection, a fit young person will take about a week to improve. Bacterial pleurisy also responds to modern medical treatment—a far cry from the days when pleurisy was a killer, particularly of children.

My father had to have some fluid removed from his chest with a needle. Was this fluid anything to do with pleurisy?

It sounds as if your father had a pleural effusion, in which the fluid comes from the pleural cavity and is lost from an inflamed surface of the pleura. Pleural effusions are just one type of pleurisy. Doctors tend to make a distinction in terminology: they call an illness that gives pain on deep breathing pleurisy, and refer to a pleural effusion, which often involves no chest pain, as just that.

Inflammation of the membrane that lines the lungs was once feared as a potentially fatal disease. Owing to advances in medical treatment, however, it can be controlled by the use of antibiotics.

Pleurisy is the name given to inflammation of the pleura, the delicate lining membrane of the lungs. It can be associated with all sorts of diseases, from serious to very minor.

In the past, mention of pleurisy alarmed people. This was because it was invariably associated with lobar pneumonia, which commonly killed young children. Nowadays, however, lobar pneumonia can be controlled with antibiotics.

The pleura

Each lung is surrounded by a lining membrane called the visceral pleura. It lines the whole lung on each side; it even lines both sides of the fissures (cracks) that divide the lung up into its various lobes.

THE PLEURA LINING THE LUNGS

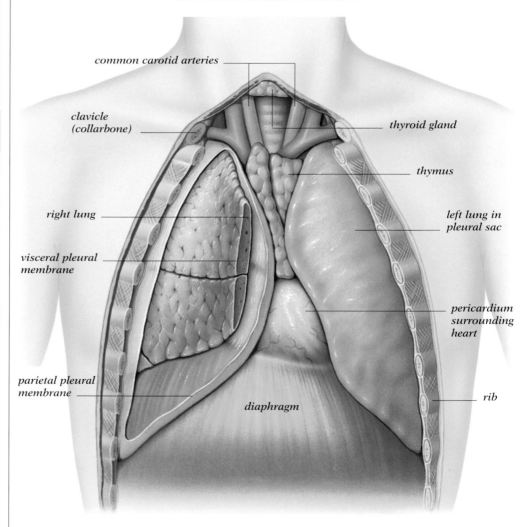

common carotid arteries

clavicle (collarbone)

thyroid gland

thymus

right lung

left lung in pleural sac

visceral pleural membrane

pericardium surrounding heart

parietal pleural membrane

diaphragm

rib

▲ *The lungs are surrounded by two layers of pleura: visceral and parietal. Pleurisy occurs when the pleura are inflamed or the space between the layers is filled with fluid.*

As this sheet of visceral pleura leaves the lung surface at each hilum (the roof of the lung at the point where the bronchus joins it), it forms another sheet, the parietal pleura, which spreads around the inside of the chest wall and the upper half of the diaphragm on one side of the chest (see Diaphragm).

In healthy people the visceral and parietal layers of pleura are always in contact with each other, and they slide over each other as the lungs move in the act of breathing. However, there is some space between the two layers. In healthy people this potential space is minimal—just enough to accommodate tiny amounts of fluid that help lubricate the two layers as they glide over each other. In one manifestation of pleurisy, however, the space can fill up with large amounts of fluid; this is called a pleural effusion.

Unlike the lung, the pleura is sensitive to pain, and it is this pain that is characteristic of pleurisy. Inflammation makes the surface of the pleura raw, and pain arises as the visceral and parietal pleura slide past each other in the process of breathing.

Who gets pleurisy?

Pleurisy can attack people of all ages, from children to the very aged. When it is caused by viral infection, it is a disease that doctors tend to associate with young people. When it is associated with pneumonia, it is generally considered to be a disease of older people. A pleural effusion may occur for a variety of reasons. This, too, tends to affect older people.

Causes

Viruses are a common cause of pleurisy. They may cause the pleural membranes to become inflamed and sore in the same way as they affect the membranes of the nose when a person has a cold. Like any other sort of viral infection, pleurisy can occur in small epidemics (see Viruses).

The symptoms of this type of pleurisy are painful chest muscles and pain on breathing. The condition usually settles down without treatment and does not give rise to complications.

Bacteria can also produce pleurisy, although they usually do this as a result of underlying pneumonia (see Bacteria). As infection spreads through the lung tissue, it eventually leads to inflammation of the outer surface of the lung. This inflammation then leads to the symptoms of pleurisy.

Bacteria can cause pleurisy in tuberculosis, a disease that is again on the increase—because of AIDS. It causes a big pleural effusion, and the painful breathing so typical of many sorts of pleurisy is not nearly as common in cases related to tuberculosis.

Another common cause of pleural effusion is cancer. Lung cancer as well as cancer from other parts of the body can spread to the pleura. If the pleura is involved, the cancer usually is inoperable (see Cancer).

Occasionally, a pleural effusion turns out to be due to neither an infection nor a tumor, but some other disease. For example, diseases that set up a general level of inflammation in the body as a result of disturbances in the body's immune system can cause a pleural effusion (see Immune System). One such disease is called systemic lupus erythematosus (see Lupus).

There is also a very rare hereditary disease that occurs almost exclusively in Armenian and Sephardic Jewish families. It is called familial Mediterranean fever, and it involves repeated attacks of inflammation in all the membranes of the lung as well as in the

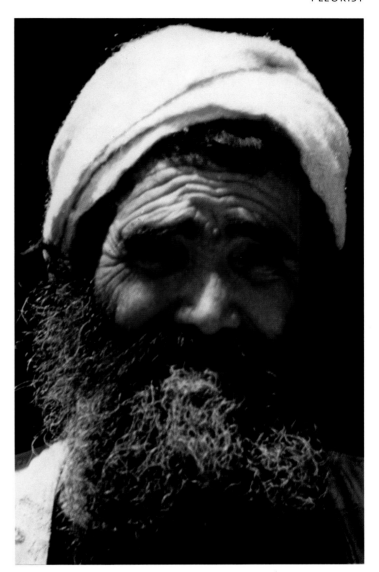

▲ *Sephardic Jews are among the principal sufferers from a rare hereditary disease called familial Mediterranean fever, which involves inflammation of the pleura.*

peritoneum (the membrane that covers the wall of the abdomen; see Peritoneum) and the pericardium (the membrane that surrounds the heart).

Perhaps the most serious pleural problem is called pulmonary embolism. In this condition, a clot—which may have formed in the leg, for example—breaks off, travels through the heart, and gets stuck in the lung. This may cause typical pleural pain, since the affected area of the lung becomes inflamed and the inflammation spreads to the pleura. Pulmonary embolisms can be fatal, but if a definite diagnosis has been made, doctors can prescribe anticoagulant drugs to stop further clots from forming.

Symptoms

The typical symptom of pleurisy is pain in the chest. This is made worse by breathing, particularly deep breathing, since the two inflamed pleural surfaces rub against each other. Shifting position may also cause pain.

I had an attack of pleurisy about six months ago. It was very unpleasant, and I am worried that it may have made me prone to repeated attacks. Is this likely?

No. Pleurisy is usually the result of an acute chest infection, such as bronchitis or pneumonia, which, once it has been treated, is completely cured and not likely to return. It is, of course, possible for you to develop another chest infection at a later date. Should you get any further chest pain, it would be wise to see your doctor about it so that he can reexamine your chest and possibly order an X ray to determine the cause of the trouble.

A few weeks ago, I fell and hit my chest on the corner of a table. Now it hurts when I breathe. Have I got pleurisy as a result of the accident?

No. It is much more likely that you injured your ribs when you fell, and, since your ribs move slightly when you breathe, this is probably why you experience pain similar to that of pleurisy.

A few weeks ago, I had a bad pain in my chest that was much worse when I coughed or took a deep breath. I was certain it was pleurisy, but my doctor insisted it wasn't. What could it have been?

Understandably, people think that any pain in the chest is likely to be due to pleurisy. There are, however, many possible causes, the majority of them a great deal more common than pleurisy. The most common cause of pain is inflammation of the muscles in the chest wall. Obviously, since the muscles are used every time you breathe, the pain will be felt when you take a particularly deep breath or when you cough. When this is the cause of pain in the chest, one particular part of the chest wall is usually tender, a symptom that does not normally occur with pleurisy. Chest pain caused by pleurisy is more likely to be felt at the sides or back of the chest than in the center.

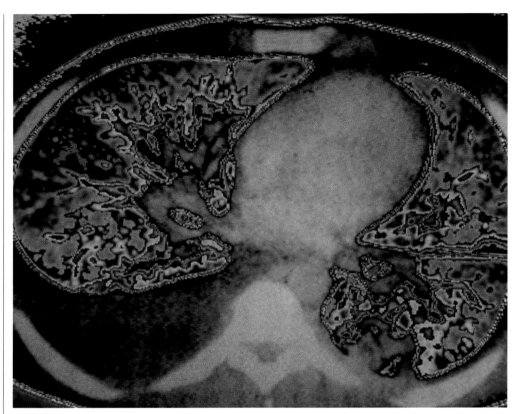

▲ *A false-color CT scan of the lungs of a patient with a right pleural effusion. The dark purple area behind the right lung (left-hand side of image) indicates a large amount of fluid. The condition is relieved by draining the fluid.*

When fluid begins to collect in the pleural space, the inflamed layers of pleura are separated, and the pain may disappear. Therefore, with a large pleural effusion, the main problem is likely to be breathlessness rather than pain.

A doctor can diagnose pleurisy by listening to a patient's description of the pain. The doctor will be helped in the diagnosis if he or she can hear what is called a "pleural rub" through the stethoscope. A pleural rub is exactly that: the sound of the two inflamed layers of pleura rubbing against each other. Each breath sounds rather like a foot crunching on packed snow. Chest X rays are also helpful, particularly when patients are suffering from pleural effusions (see X Rays).

Treatment

The type of treatment prescribed will depend on the underlying condition. Pleuritic symptoms can be very painful, and can require a painkiller, usually aspirin, which relieves pain and also reduces inflammation (see Painkillers).

When a large amount of fluid is present, it has to be drained. The procedure is simple: the doctor freezes a small section of the chest with local anesthetic, and then passes a needle into the pleural space to draw off the fluid (see Local Anesthetics). By using a special needle the doctor can also remove a piece of the pleura for examination under a microscope. This will be useful if the diagnosis is not clear.

Outlook

The outlook for a patient suffering from pleurisy depends on the underlying condition. Pleurisy itself presents very few dangers, although when it is due to a fast-growing tumor, for example, it is obviously a serious condition (see Tumors). The outlook is excellent, however, in the case of a healthy person who gets an isolated attack of pleurisy as the result of a virus.

See also: Antibiotics; Breathing; Chest; Inflammation; Lung and lung diseases; Membranes; Pneumonia; Pulmonary disorders; Stethoscope; Tuberculosis

Pneumoconiosis

Questions and Answers

Could I get pneumoconiosis from exposure to other people's cigarette smoke?

No. Pneumoconiosis is brought about by contact with mineral dust—the sort of dust that you would find in a mine or in a stone quarry. If you have never been exposed to this sort of dust, you are not at risk. However, cigarette smoke will make the disease worse once it has become established.

Do you get different types of pneumoconiosis depending on the sort of dust you have been exposed to?

Yes; the type will be evident from a chest X ray and show up as a fine speckling, whether or not there are symptoms. With coal miners, there may be no symptoms, or very few. The changes in the lungs will vary according to the type of coal being mined.

My uncle was a sandblaster and he died from lung disease. Could he have had pneumoconiosis?

Probably. Before World War II, sandblasting was a well-known cause of pneumoconiosis. In sandblasting, metal is cleaned by blowing sand on it at very high speed. Sand contains a lot of silicone, and silicone dust seems to cause many problems in the lungs. Today, strict safety precautions are applied if this technique is used.

Do all coal miners get pneumoconiosis?

No. It depends on the type of coal that is being mined, since some types are more likely to cause problems than others. In Wales, for instance, an estimated 3 to 15 percent of coal miners were affected, usually to a small extent; in the United States the estimate varies between 4 and 45 percent.

Pneumoconiosis is a debilitating lung disease caused by inhaling mineral dust. It is a particular hazard for miners and quarry workers, but precautions to reduce the dust levels in these occupations can be very effective.

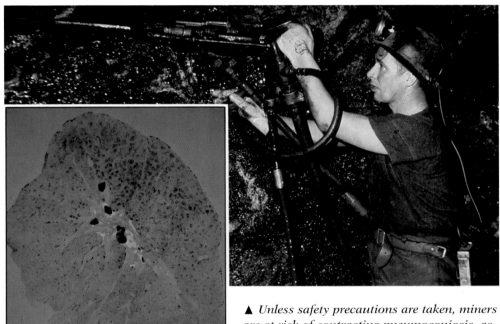

▲ *Unless safety precautions are taken, miners are at risk of contracting pneumoconiosis, as shown in the section of lung tissue inset.*

The air people breathe contains particles of dust. Dust does not usually cause any problems, although excessive exposure may contribute to chronic bronchitis. However, when dust of mineral origin is breathed in, the lung tissue reacts in an abnormal way, and this results in pneumoconiosis. The severity of the disease depends on the concentration of dust in the air that is breathed in.

Coal dust is the most common cause of pneumoconiosis, but other forms of dust can also give rise to the disease. Silica dust, which occurs in quarrying and in industries that use a lot of quartz, can give rise to a form of the disease called silicosis.

Pneumoconiosis may lead to emphysema, a disease in which the air sacs in the lungs (alveoli) and the narrow passages leading to them (bronchioles) become permanently distended with air. Pneumoconiosis alone may not cause any symptoms; the emphysema that develops causes many of the symptoms. Smoking is an important aggravating factor (see Smoking).

Symptoms and dangers

The main symptom of pneumoconiosis is breathlessness, which can vary in severity. On an X ray, the lung changes will appear as a fine speckling, but the picture varies according to the type of dust causing the disease (see X Rays).

Pneumoconiosis can sometimes be rapidly progressive and the amount of lung destruction very great. This leads to extensive scarring of the lung with fibrous tissue (massive pulmonary fibrosis).

Outlook and prevention

Pneumoconiosis cannot be cured, but treatment can alleviate symptoms. Prevention is thus vital and requires careful control of dust and wearing masks at work. People at risk should be X-rayed regularly and their jobs changed at the first sign of disease. Smoking must be discouraged.

See also: Bronchitis; Emphysema; Lung and lung diseases; Occupational hazards; Pulmonary disorders; Silicosis

Pneumonia

Pneumonia—acute inflammation of the lungs—used to be one of the great killers, attacking the young and fit almost as readily as the aged and infirm. Treatment with antibiotics has now made it possible to save countless lives.

Questions and Answers

Is double pneumonia worse than the ordinary type of pneumonia?

In the past, one of the most common forms of pneumonia was lobar pneumonia, in which one complete lobe of one of the lungs became infected, usually with the pneumococcus bacterium. (There are three lobes on the right lung, two on the left.) In double pneumonia, more than one lung was infected; this was obviously a more serious condition than involvement of only a single lung. Pneumonias involving more than one lung have a higher mortality than those that are confined to a single lung.

When my father had pneumonia he received treatment from a physical therapist that involved hitting him on the chest. What good could this have done him?

The physical therapist is vital in the treatment of pneumonia to ensure that all the infected secretions of the inflamed mucous membranes are brought up from the depths of the lungs and coughed up. Thumping the chest wall is one technique that a physical therapist will use to loosen the secretions, and some patients find that it brings relief from breathlessness. However, it does not affect the rate of recovery from the pneumonia.

Does pneumonia tend to be worse in people who suffer from asthma?

The main problem in people who suffer from asthma is that their bronchial tubes tend to become constricted (narrowed) easily. Any infection in the chest will increase this problem; there doesn't have to be full-blown pneumonia for someone to get a bad asthmatic attack. However, when an asthmatic does have pneumonia, it will definitely tend to constrict the bronchial tubes, and this will make the condition worse.

Pneumonia usually occurs as a result of a bacterial infection, but it may also arise from a viral or fungal infection or from inhaling foreign matter into the lungs. Owing to treatment with antibiotics, fewer people now die of pneumonia (see Antibiotics). However, the aged, people with chronic lung disorders, and those already weakened by other diseases remain at risk.

Causes

To understand how pneumonia affects the lungs, it is important to look at their structure. The breathing tube that supplies air to the lungs is the windpipe (trachea). This splits into two branches (the bronchi), which in turn divide into three main branches on the right and two main branches on the left. Each of these branches supplies one lobe of one of the lungs: there are three lobes on the right and two on the left, separated from each other by thin membranes of fibrous tissue. Each

LOBAR PNEUMONIA

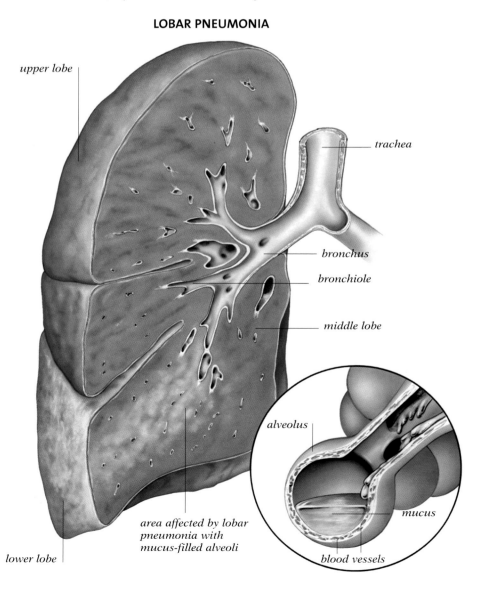

upper lobe

trachea

bronchus

bronchiole

middle lobe

alveolus

mucus

area affected by lobar pneumonia with mucus-filled alveoli

lower lobe

blood vessels

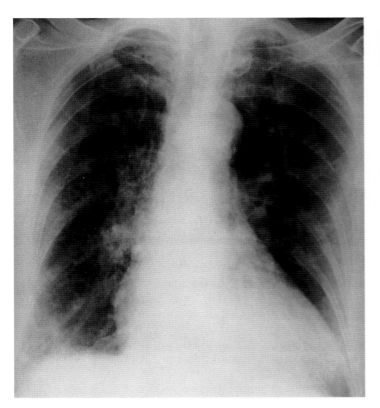

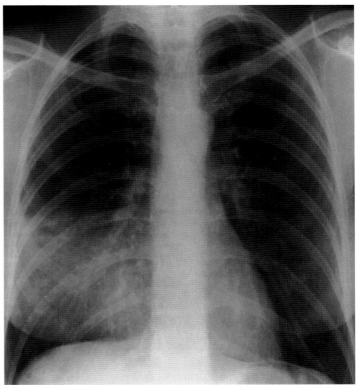

of the main bronchi then splits down into finer branches that supply all of the tiny air sacs (alveoli) where oxygen finally crosses from the air inside the lungs into the blood.

When the chest is infected, the lung tissue becomes inflamed. If the inflammation is confined to the bronchi it is called bronchitis, and it results in a thickening of the membrane that lines the bronchi and the production of large amounts of secretions from the glands in the bronchi (see Bronchitis).

In pneumonia, the infection occurs in the smaller bronchi (the bronchioli) and the alveoli, which become solid with secretions, rather than filled with air. This process is called consolidation. On a chest X ray the affected area shows up as a white patch, rather than as the black area that would be seen in healthy lung tissue (see X Rays). The congestion of the lungs may severely affect breathing.

There are two main types of pneumonia. Lobar pneumonia was, in the past, the more common of the two. It is nearly always caused by the pneumococcus bacterium. Only one lobe of the lung tends to be involved, and this lobe becomes consolidated while the rest of the lung remains relatively normal.

Bronchopneumonia can be caused by many different sorts of organisms, but usually one of several bacteria is responsible, the most common of which is the *Haemophilus influenzae* bacterium. Other kinds of bacteria that can cause bronchopneumonia include the pneumococcus and the staphylococcus. Staphylococcus is the more serious. This kind of bronchopneumonia tends to appear after

▲ *A chest X ray reveals the type of pneumonia. Bronchopneumonia (above left) is distinguished by white patches on all or part of a lung; note those on the right lung (left-hand side of image). Lobar pneumonia (above right), involves the whole lobe.*

▼ *Bronchopneumonia caused by the pneumococcus bacterium.*

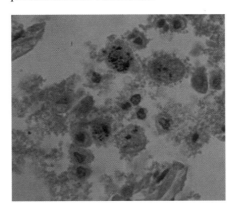

an attack of flu, and may cause death even in people who were previously healthy.

Bronchopneumonia is characterized by small patches of consolidation that appear all over the lungs. These patches may be concentrated in one lung, or even in one part of one lung, but a whole lobe is not involved. Bronchopneumonia can occur at the same time as bronchitis, and it often results when bronchitis spreads to involve the rest of the lung tissue. This frequently happens to people who have chronic (long-term) chest problems, but it is also common for people to get acute bronchopneumonia in addition to chronic bronchitis.

Viruses can cause pneumonia, but more often a primary viral infection in the upper part of the respiratory tract (the throat and nose) is followed by a secondary bacterial infection in the lungs (see Viruses).

Other microscopic organisms, such as chlamydia (which causes psittacosis, a disease caught from caged birds), rickettsia (which causes typhus and Q fever), and mycoplasma (a funguslike organism), can also cause pneumonia (see Q Fever; Typhus). People with AIDS are particularly likely to develop a severe pneumonia caused by the organism *Pneumocystis carinii* (see AIDS).

Pneumonia may also arise as a result of a blockage of one of the main bronchial tubes, for instance from cancer of the bronchus (see Cancer). Similarly, chronic disorders of the bronchus, such as bronchiectasis (in which the bronchi continually produce pus as a result of a chronic infection that also destroys the normal bronchial

Questions and Answers

Can people's lungs be permanently damaged by pneumonia?

Yes. Some of the bacteria that cause pneumonia, such as the staphylococcus, can lead to the formation of abscesses that remain as a scar even after treatment. However, most cases of pneumonia can now be treated with antibiotics and recovery of the lungs is complete.

I've heard that a simple cold that spreads to the chest can cause pneumonia. Is this true?

Yes, infections in the upper part of the respiratory tract—the nose and throat—can be a cause of pneumonia. The original infection is usually due to a virus, but as a result of this a bacterium can become established lower down in the chest, causing pneumonia.

Are inhalations with steam good for people who have pneumonia?

Inhalations with steam, or with a substance called tincture of benzoin, were used much more in the past than they are today. However, they may very well make people cough up infected phlegm and feel better. A more modern form of inhalation is with drugs that widen the bronchial tubes. These are given as a vapor through an oxygen mask.

Why are elderly people more prone to pneumonia?

Anyone who is weak, either through age or through illness, will be prone to pneumonia, and for this reason it is often what finally leads to the death of people who are already ill with some other disease. The resistance of the body to infection is reduced, and once pneumonia has become established, an elderly patient may be too weak to cough up all the infected secretions, so that the infection becomes worse. This leads to a further weakening of the patient, who then has even less ability to clear the sputum.

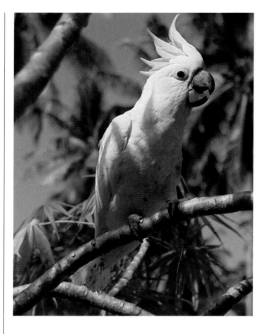

▲ *Though beautiful to look at, the cockatoo may transmit the chlamydia virus, which causes psittacosis—a type of pneumonia. However, it is fairly uncommon.*

How to prevent pneumonia

Stop smoking, especially if you have long-standing chest trouble.

If pneumonia is prevalent in your area and you are at high risk, ask your doctor to immunize you against influenza.

If you have lung disease, ask your doctor to immunize you against pneumococcus.

Don't wait for a chest ailment to get better on its own; seek medical attention immediately.

Avoid crowds during the flu season.

Keep up a high level of nutrition and health—all types of pneumonia pose the worst threat to the weak, the elderly, and people who are debilitated.

wall), can produce pneumonia by blocking the tubes and allowing pus to be sucked back into normal lung tissue (see Pus).

Finally, pneumonia can result from inhaling foreign objects, such as loose teeth or peanuts, into the lungs. This is called aspiration pneumonia. However, the main kind of aspiration pneumonia occurs as a result of unconsciousness, because when a person is unconscious the coughing mechanism that normally prevents food and other foreign substances from going down the wrong way is absent (see Unconsciousness). Therefore, it is important for unconscious patients to be watched carefully so that no such inhalations occur, for example, when general anesthesia is given (see Anesthetics), or when emergency resuscitation is needed (see Resuscitation).

Symptoms

The main symptom of pneumonia is a cough, which varies according to the type of condition. In bronchopneumonia with added acute bronchitis, infected (yellow or green) sputum may be produced; in a viral pneumonia there could be a dry cough with no sputum at all.

In bronchopneumonia there is usually a cough, although it is not the main symptom. Lobar pneumonia is characterized by fever, and unless the patient is treated with antibiotics, he or she will have a very high temperature. Since the whole lobe is involved, the inflammation may spread to the lining of the pleura, causing pleurisy, which will result in the additional symptom of pain on coughing or on taking a deep breath.

In bronchopneumonia caused by bacteria, the symptoms tend to vary according to how much extra bronchitis there is. However, there is nearly always more sputum produced in bronchopneumonia than in lobar pneumonia, and pleurisy is a less common occurrence. The patient usually has a raised temperature, but it is not as high as in lobar pneumonia.

Bronchopneumonia is more likely to affect older people and those who are sick or infirm. Often there are fewer symptoms in older

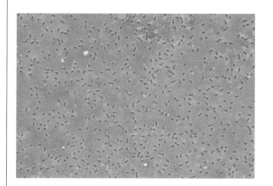

▲ *In lobar pneumonia, a sputum sample examined under a microscope will reveal the presence of pneumococcal bacteria.*

Causes and treatment of pneumonia

TYPE	CAUSE	SYMPTOMS	TREATMENT
PNEUMONIAS CAUSED BY A BACTERIUM			
Lobar pneumonia	Pneumococcus bacterium	Cough, pain on breathing, fever. Rust-colored sputum.	Antibiotics
Bronchopneumonia	Various organisms, particularly *Haemophilus influenzae*	Cough is the main symptom, but there may also be fever. Green or yellow sputum.	Antibiotics appropriate to the organism concerned
Pneumonia leading to abscess formation	Staphylococcus and klebsiella bacteria; anaerobic bacteria	A severe feverish illness with a cough	Antibiotics
Aspiration pneumonia	Various organisms. As a result of inhalation, usually while patient is unconscious.	Fever and cough. Often causes lung abscess.	Antibiotics
PNEUMONIAS NOT CAUSED BY A BACTERIUM			
Viral pneumonia	Chicken pox, influenza	Cough and fever without much sputum being produced	Antibiotics if the lungs then become infected by a bacterium. Ventilation on a respirator may be required.
	Respiratory syncytial virus	Occurs in newborn babies. Causes breathlessness.	
Pneumocystis carinii pneumonia	Immune deficiency allowing infection with *P. carinii*	Slight fever, weakness, breathlessness, and cyanosis	The drug pentamidine isethionate
Q fever	Rickettsia virus	Cough and fever, not much sputum	Tetracycline or erythromycin
Mycoplasma	Very small fungal organisms, similar to bacteria, but with no thick cell wall	Cough and fever, not much sputum	Tetracycline or erythromycin

people than in people who are young and fit, even though when the disease occurs in older people, it may cause death after a long illness.

In the rare forms of pneumonia caused by organisms other than bacteria, the symptoms vary, but by and large, fever is common. Changes in the lungs are obvious in X rays; the cough and sputum production are less than in bacterial pneumonia.

Dangers and complications

One of the most common complications of all kinds of pneumonia is pleurisy. This may lead to a pleural effusion (a collection of fluid within the pleural cavity). If this fluid then becomes infected, it leads to pus formation in the pleural cavity, causing emphysema.

Pockets of pus can also form within the lung, causing a lung abscess. This is especially likely to develop in staphylococcal pneumonia and in a rare form of lobar pneumonia called klebsiella, as well as with pneumonia caused by anaerobic bacteria (bacteria that do not need oxygen to survive). Lung abscesses are a serious problem and occur only as a result of severe lung infection (see Abscess).

In general, though, rather than giving rise to other complications, pneumonia is a complication of other diseases. It is for this reason that pneumonia, usually severe bronchopneumonia, may be fatal, because it is so often the final event in the life of someone who is already very weak, sick, or aged.

Treatment

In fit people, treatment with antibiotics is generally all that is necessary. However, in older people, or people who already have a chronic chest disease or another illness, it is important to make sure that the secretions in the lung produced by pneumonia are coughed up and not allowed to remain in the chest, where they can cause further problems. The physical therapist has a vital role to play in helping people with pneumonia to clear these secretions (see Physical Therapy). Drugs that are inhaled as a vapor through an oxygen mask may help to widen the bronchi, which tend to narrow in pneumonia.

Outlook

The outlook in pneumonia depends on the age and state of health of the patient. A young, fit person who gets lobar pneumonia should make a total and rapid recovery, whereas an aged person with chronic bronchitis who has probably already had a number of attacks of bronchopneumonia is at some risk of dying if he or she has a further attack. Pneumonia in someone who is very weak as a result of disease can be fatal, even with antibiotic treatment.

See also: **Bacteria; Breathing; Chest; Coughing; Lung and lung diseases; Pleurisy; Psittacosis; Staphylococcus**

Podiatry

Foot disorders cause a great deal of pain and sometimes disability. Qualified podiatrists can diagnose and treat a wide range of problems and give advice on how to keep the feet healthy and pain-free.

What is an ingrown toenail, and how should it be treated?

The name is misleading; the toenail does not always grow in. Swollen inflamed tissue along the nail edge can move over the edge of the nail, producing a deceptive appearance. The condition is very painful, and it is usually caused by cutting the toenails in a curve and down at the sides (rather than straight across at the end) or by wearing tight shoes. A podiatrist will be able to treat it by removing the edge of the nail, along with any nail splinters, using a local anesthetic. He or she will then clean and dry the area and apply an antiseptic, then sterile cotton or gauze, a sterile dressing, and finally tubular gauze.

I was sick recently and had to spend a lot of time in bed. Now that I'm able to get up, my feet are flat and painful to walk on. Will they stay like this?

No. This is a temporary condition. Because you have not been using the muscles in your feet, they have become flabby and weak and cannot support the arches. A podiatrist can give you some foot exercises to do every day that will strengthen the muscles and help to gradually build up the arches.

I do a lot of running, but recently I have had a pain in the ball of my foot that gets worse whenever I run. What could be causing this?

It may be a fracture in one or more of your foot bones (metatarsals). Running subjects the feet to repeated stress, and this can cause fractures called "march fractures," which produce pain in the ball of the foot that gets worse after any prolonged exertion. The diagnosis can be confirmed by X ray. If it is a fracture, your foot will need to be strapped in, and you will need to rest it for at least a few weeks until the fracture has repaired itself.

Podiatry is the diagnosis and treatment of feet and their ailments. It is unusual for everyday foot problems to be treated by physicians or surgeons. Instead, they are dealt with by podiatrists who have had specialized training. In addition to examining the feet and applying dressings, podiatrists perform minor surgical procedures using local anesthesia and identify those patients who do need to be treated by a physician or surgeon.

The most common disorders that podiatrists deal with can be put into three basic categories: those that arise from biomechanical factors, those caused by infection, and those caused by general disease. As a person gets older, existing problems may get worse and new ones can develop.

Biomechanical disorders

The feet have two main functions: to support the weight of the body and to act as a lever to move the body forward when a person walks or runs. Many demands are placed on the feet, from the fine balance required by a ballet dancer to the propulsion required by an athlete (see Balance; Movement). These extremes of activity, in addition to the more common everyday activities, place mechanical stresses on the feet. Abnormal or excessive stress—for example, as a result of bearing heavy weight or wearing inappropriate footwear—can cause foot disorders. Bearing heavy weight does not just mean carrying heavy loads; it is also a problem for obese people (see Obesity; Weight). One of the best ways of avoiding stress-related foot problems is to wear comfortable shoes that fit properly. Narrow or pointed shoes, high heels, platform soles, and shoes that do not hold the feet in place can cause all kinds of problems.

Flat feet

When babies are first born, they appear to have flat feet, but the arches develop as the tendons, muscles, and ligaments get stronger with use. If the arch of the foot does not develop or if it disappears, then the condition known as flat feet occurs. The feet can become flat if the whole

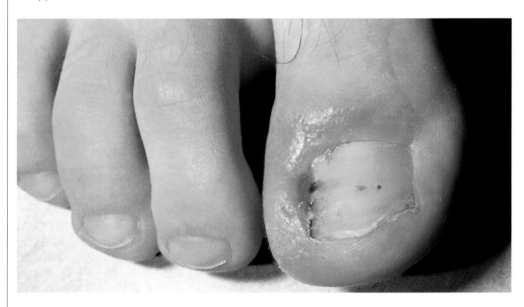

▲ *This patient has an infection of the soft tissue alongside the edge of the large toenail. The swelling of the skin extends a little way across the nail edge, producing an appearance that misleadingly suggests an ingrown nail.*

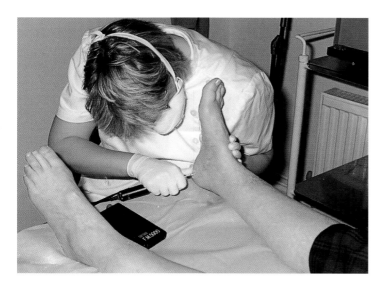

▲ *Sometimes the podiatrist uses a machine to file down calluses—areas of thickened skin caused by prolonged pressure or friction—on a patient's feet.*

structure of the arch collapses. This type of flat foot does not usually cause any pain or discomfort and is nothing to worry about, though an individual may find that his or her shoes wear unevenly. The cause of flat feet is poorly understood. This condition involves the loss of both the front-to-back arch and the side-to-side arch. It can cause pain and discomfort in the feet and also in the ankles, knees, and lower back, because the loss of the arches affects the way that a person stands and walks. Podiatrists treat patients with this type of flat feet by using special inserts for the shoes, called orthoses; the type of orthosis will depend on individual differences in flattening. Sometimes the shoes may need to be modified.

Bunions
A bunion is an abnormal enlargement at the outside edge of the joint between the foot and the base of the big toe and is a very common disorder. The joint, which is often swollen and tender, points outward at a sharp angle, while the big toe points inward. The other toes become affected and corns can develop, because the deformity causes increased stress on other parts of the feet.

Bunions tend to develop in people with an inherited weakness in the toe joints. A bunion is made worse by badly fitting shoes, especially shoes with high heels and pointed toes, so it is not surprising that more women than men are affected. Once the deformity has started, it tends to get worse and will not correct itself, even if shoes are not worn.

If a bunion is painful, a person should see a podiatrist, who will remove any corns that have developed and give treatment to relieve the pain. This may include protective padding to ease the pressure on the joint; shoe alterations, such as a balloon patch on the side of the shoe; or an appliance, such as a shield, that fits over the tender joint and protects it (see Dressings and Bandages).

Corns and calluses
Corns and calluses are areas of skin that become thickened by constant pressure, often caused by new shoes or shoes that do not fit properly; and once corns and calluses have developed, pressure on them causes tenderness in the tissues underneath. Corns are small and develop on the toes, whereas calluses are larger and develop on the soles of the feet. Wearing high heels can also cause calluses, since this type of shoe puts more pressure on the ball of the foot. Some people have a natural tendency to develop calluses because their skin is delicate.

The podiatrist will remove the thickened skin of a callus with a scalpel, then apply an antiseptic and a padded dressing. If the skin is dry, the podiatrist will probably recommend that an emollient be applied twice a day to soften the skin and prevent further calluses. With corns, the podiatrist will remove the nucleus with a scalpel, and as with calluses, an emollient should be applied.

Infections
Foot infections may be caused by bacteria, viruses, or fungi. Bacterial infections are not very common, but if a person does get one, the podiatrist will prescribe either an antiseptic, if the infection is mild, or an antibiotic, if it is more severe or persistent. Some groups of people are more prone to bacterial infections: these include older people, particularly those with poor circulation; people with certain medical conditions, including diabetes mellitus; those with poor nutrition or anemia; and those who are taking certain medicines such as corticosteroids and immunosuppressive or cytotoxic drugs.

Verrucae (warts)
The most common viral infection is a plantar wart—a type of wart on the sole of the foot, commonly known as a verruca. The virus enters a skin cell, where it multiplies and spreads to adjacent cells. The hard, horny swelling this produces usually gets pushed under the skin by standing and walking, and so may irritate the sensitive nerve endings and cause pain. Most people catch verrucae at swimming pools, since the virus finds it easier to get into the skin cells when they are wet.

If a verruca develops, it is advisable to wear rubber shoes for swimming; at home, a personal bath mat and towel should be used so that the virus does not spread to other family members. A verruca does not always cause pain, and if it is left alone, it will usually disappear within six to eight months. If it lasts much longer than this or is painful, a podiatrist should be consulted.

There are no effective drugs that can kill the verruca virus, so treatment of verrucae involves killing the skin cells that contain the virus. Most podiatrists do this by using either chemical cautery, cryotherapy, or electrosurgery.

Methods of removal
Chemical cautery is effective, produces rapid results, and is not usually painful. The podiatrist will apply a caustic chemical, taking care not to spread it onto the surrounding healthy tissue. A circular pad with a hole in the middle is placed over the verruca and covered with a zinc oxide plaster. After about seven days, the podiatrist will remove the dead tissue from the foot, and if the verruca has not been completely destroyed, he or she will apply more of the caustic chemical and a fresh dressing.

In cryotherapy, the infected tissue is cooled to very low temperatures. This causes ice crystals to form in the fluid inside and around the cells, and the cells then rupture. The temperature in the tissues must be reduced to at least −4°F (−20°C) for the treatment to be effective. It is a technique that requires only a single treatment, but it can be painful.

I work in a store on Saturdays, and my feet are often aching by the end of the day. Why is this?

Aching feet are a very common problem. Standing for a long time, doing a lot of walking, and being overweight can all make your feet ache. The pain happens because the supporting muscles get tired, and the ligaments become stretched through supporting the load on the arches. A podiatrist will apply a figure-eight strapping to your foot and ankle to relieve the symptoms, and he or she will advise you on the type of shoes you should wear to give your feet the firm support that they need.

My second toe is bent into an inverted "V" shape and rubs on my shoes. Is there anything I can do about it?

This is a common complaint called hammertoe. You should wear shoes deep enough to remove the pressure on the joint, and padding will help to relieve the pain. Your podiatrist can give you a splint to straighten the toes.

Why does my podiatrist look at my shoes whenever I visit him?

Your podiatrist will check your shoes for size, shape, style, suitability, and also any signs of abnormal wear on the heels, soles, and tops. Abnormal wear on the soles or heels, or distortion of the tops, may indicate certain foot disorders, and this inspection will help to diagnose the problem.

I am training to be a ballet dancer. I have constant problems with my feet, especially bunions. What can I do to prevent or reduce the effects of strain on my toes?

It is important for you to see a podiatrist regularly, especially if you are planning to have a career in ballet. The podiatrist will check to see that your ballet slippers fit correctly and will advise you on general foot care.

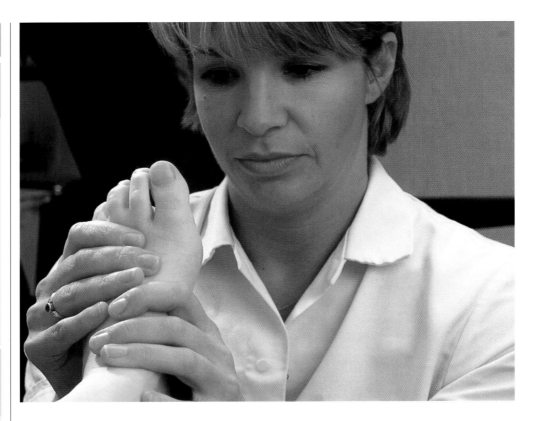

▲ *A podiatrist presses and manipulates the foot of a patient during an examination. Problems treated may include bunions, hammertoes, and foot ulcers.*

Electrosurgery is also a single treatment technique that destroys the tissue by heat. If the podiatrist is using this method, the patient will be given a local anesthetic, as there may be a little pain (see Anesthetics).

Fungal infections

Other problems that are associated with wearing shoes are fungal infections. These infections are common, because shoes help to create the warm, moist conditions between the toes in which fungi thrive. The fungi digest the dead skin that the body sheds each day and can also cause inflammation and damage to living skin cells—in severe cases, they can infect the toenails.

Fungal infections can be treated with an antifungal paint or ointment, which should be applied twice daily until two or three weeks after the symptoms disappear. If the toenails are infected, they may take up to 18 months to clear. The best way to prevent fungal infections from recurring is to wash the feet at least once a day and dry them thoroughly, especially between the toes. Antifungal powders can also be used inside the shoes. The most common antifungal drugs used to treat fungal infections of the feet are the azole group, especially the imidazole and triazole drugs.

General diseases

Older people and those who have diseases that cause reduced sensation in the feet or diseases that affect the circulation, such as diabetes mellitus and peripheral artery disease, should take special care of their feet and should never neglect any cuts or sores that do develop (see Arteries and Artery Disease; Diabetes). Cuts and sores take longer to heal in people with poor circulation than in healthy people and can become seriously infected without attention from a podiatrist.

Diseases such as arthritis, in addition to affecting the joints in the feet, can make it difficult for people to reach their feet, and this can also be a problem as people get older (see Arthritis). If this is the case, a podiatrist should be visited on a regular basis so that he or she can cut the toenails and treat any minor problems before they develop into more serious ones.

See also: Bacteria; Bunions; Corns; Feet; Fractures; Ingrown toenail; Nails; Verruca; Viruses; Warts

Poisoning

Questions and Answers

Do all poisons cause deep unconsciousness in the victim?

No. Tranquilizers and sleeping tablets will lead to coma when taken in an overdose, but others such as acetaminophen and aspirin can leave the patient wide awake for as long as 48 hours or more after being taken. Corrosives that burn the esophagus also leave the patient awake, so the state of consciousness is not a good guide to the severity of poisoning.

What is alcohol poisoning?

Alcohol can slowly poison the liver and cause cirrhosis, a disease that can be fatal. Large, unaccustomed amounts of alcohol taken in a short time can cause a coma or death. Alcohol can make the body susceptible to acetaminophen (Tylenol) poisoning; for this reason, most painkillers cannot be given to alcoholics. In children, alcohol, even in small amounts, can result in unconsciousness. It can also increase the effects of medicines such as tranquilizers, sleeping tablets, and pills for hay fever or motion sickness, and lead to drowsiness and unsteadiness.

What can I do to reduce my family's risk of poisoning by medicines?

If you buy medicines such as painkillers or cold remedies, ask for as few as possible. Don't get twice the amount you need "so that they'll be there for next time"; 25 tablets should be the maximum. When buying medicines for a child, tell the pharmacist this, and give the child's age. Adults' medicines should never be given to children. Prescription tablets should always be kept in childproof bottles and put away out of reach of children. Return any unused medicines to your pharmacist if a medication is changed or a course of treatment is finished.

A large number of everyday household substances contain poisons, and because they are so common, it is easy to overlook their potential dangers. Beware of carelessness, which can all too easily lead to tragedy.

Doctors consider poisoning a modern epidemic. Millions of people are accidentally poisoned every year and there are around 5,000 deaths each year from foodborne diseases alone.

Accidental cases of poisoning, either in the home or at work, are often the result of carelessness or industrial incidents. Other cases can be a result of deliberate self-poisoning; the number of such cases has increased dramatically in recent years. Whatever the cause, many of these cases can be avoided. By examining the problem and the areas of greatest risk, everyone can play a part in preventing some of these tragic events. It is vital, for instance, to be aware of the potential danger of many commonplace substances used daily in the home.

ORGANS AT RISK

▶ *Even a beneficial substance such as aspirin can have a toxic effect on the body if too much is taken. Different organs in the body are susceptible to different poisons, producing varying symptoms.*

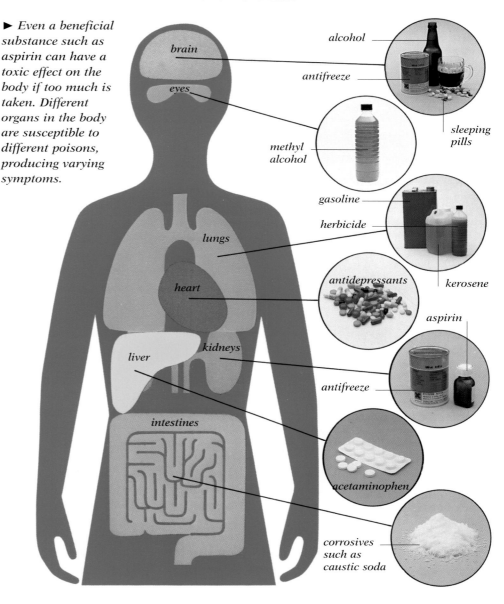

brain
eyes
alcohol
antifreeze
sleeping pills
methyl alcohol
gasoline
herbicide
antidepressants
kerosene
aspirin
lungs
heart
antifreeze
liver
kidneys
intestines
acetaminophen
corrosives such as caustic soda

Are there any aerosol sprays that are poisonous?

Most aerosols, including bug sprays, are not poisonous, or are not potentially very dangerous. An exception is oven cleaner, which contains a caustic substance that could burn the skin. With any aerosol it is important to read the manufacturer's instructions carefully to see what precautions should be taken and what the hazards are. If an aerosol is accidentally sprayed into the eye, keep the eyelid open to allow as much of the substance to evaporate as possible and wash for several minutes under a running faucet. Some aerosols can be dangerous if directly inhaled.

Can poisoning occur in people in the form of epidemics?

Yes. An epidemic of poisoning is said to occur when a single agent is responsible for poisoning a large number of people. This can occur through contaminated food or water supplies. The relevant authorities take great care to prevent this. However, in 1981, in Spain, a large epidemic of poisoning was caused by contaminated cooking oil; outbreaks on a smaller scale also occur from time to time.

Can exhaust fumes from vehicles cause poisoning?

Yes. Exhaust fumes from any type of vehicle contain the highly poisonous gas carbon monoxide, so a vehicle engine should never be left running in an unventilated space. Care should also be taken to ensure that the exhaust pipe does not leak, because, even in small amounts, the gas might build up on a long drive and cause sickness, headaches, or even death. Until recently, gasoline also contained lead compounds, which were given off in exhaust fumes. Lead can cause brain damage in high concentrations, especially in children. Leaded fuels have now been banned in many countries, including the United States.

DANGERS IN THE KITCHEN

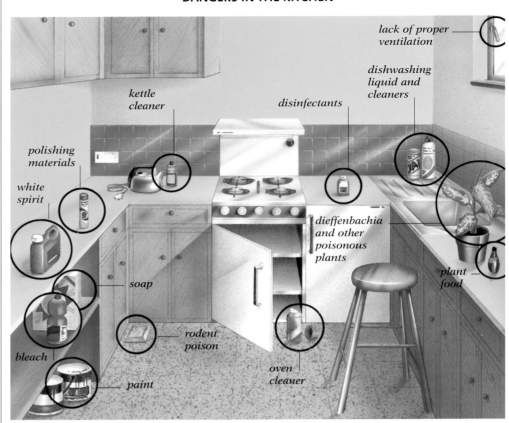

▲ *Kitchens are dangerous places for children. Many products and plants are poisonous and should be kept high up or in locked cupboards. All gas appliances need ventilation.*

Those at risk

The possibility of accidental poisoning is present throughout a person's life. However, there are certain ages when people may be particularly at risk of accidental or intentional poisoning.

When young children start to explore their surroundings, it is natural for them to put objects or liquids into their mouths, particularly if the objects are small or brightly colored. Children aged two to five years are especially at risk of poisoning by materials they find within their reach.

Teenagers often suffer emotional conflicts. Some of them seek to resolve these conflicts by taking an overdose of painkillers, sleeping tablets, or medicines that have been prescribed for their parents (see Painkillers). Their intention is very rarely to take their life. More often it is to attract attention and indirectly to seek help, or to avoid a difficult situation. Doctors and psychologists use the term "suicidal gesture" to describe this kind of behavior. However, some teenagers accidentally die because they underestimate the effects of the poisonous substances that they take.

Both suicidal gestures and genuine attempts can occur in adults who are severely depressed. In the elderly especially, suicidal intentions can be provoked by factors such as chronic illness or pain, loneliness, and depression, and poisoning is more often fatal in this age group than in any other (see Depression).

What is a poison?

It is difficult to say precisely which substances are poisonous. Even water or oxygen, when present

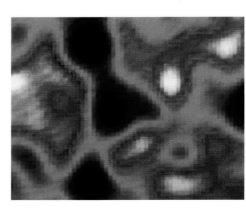

► *A scan of a brain affected by carbon monoxide, which is very poisonous, shows reduced activity in the dark blue areas.*

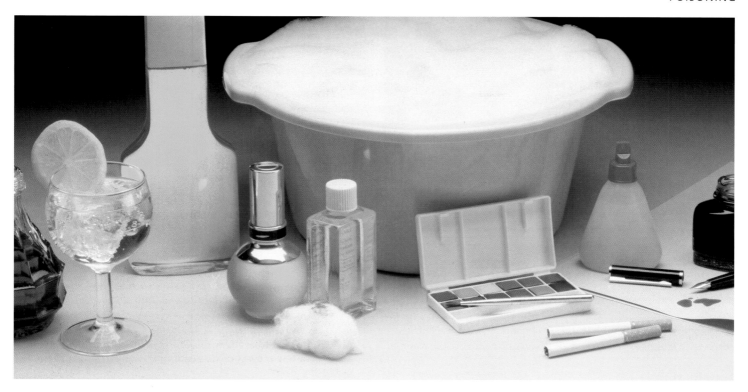

▲ *Many people do not realize the potential danger of common products. Vinegar, detergents, cigarettes, alcohol, perfume, cosmetics, ink, gum, and paints can all be lethal.*

in excess, can damage the body (see Oxygen). Also, many lifesaving medicines can be fatal when taken in large doses (see Medicines). A poison is best defined as any substance consumed in sufficient quantity to damage the normal working of the body.

Poisons include a vast range of substances that can enter the body through the skin, mouth, or lungs. They include stings by insects such as bees and wasps, and venom from poisonous fish, spiders, or snakes (see Snakebite). Gases, fumes from industrial works, vehicle exhausts, and fires can also be poisonous. Fires kill people as often by poisoning as by direct burning or lack of oxygen, since fabrics and plastics burning in enclosed spaces can rapidly produce large amounts of highly toxic fumes.

Food—particularly meat and dairy products—can cause poisoning when it has not been properly prepared or refrigerated. Food poisoning usually causes vomiting and diarrhea, which clear up in a few days but can occasionally be more serious.

Some common plants, such as deadly nightshade, yew, and laburnum, contain poisonous substances. In remote parts of the world, indigenous peoples use these natural poisons in hunting.

Many tablets, medicines, and domestic products that are commonly found in most homes can also be dangerous. As most of them will not have a warning of "poison" written on them, it is worth knowing which ones are more likely to be toxic.

How a poison acts

Poisonous substances do their damage in a variety of ways. Sleeping pills, tranquilizers, excessive alcohol, and a number of other substances can depress the working of the brain to the extent that it no longer maintains respiration; death results because oxygen is not taken in through the lungs. Some poisons act by blocking the action of vital enzymes necessary for cell function. Cyanide, for instance, inhibits certain enzymes and prevents the cells from using oxygen (see Enzymes).

Other poisons will act directly on one or more of the body's organs. For example, antidepressants can cause serious abnormal rhythms of the heart. If any type of petroleum compound is swallowed, it may pass through the system and out of the body, but if any amount reaches the lungs it can cause a type of pneumonia that is very difficult to treat (see Pneumonia). This is why a person who has swallowed gasoline, or similar oily products, should not be made to vomit: some of the vomit may be taken into the lungs.

Corrosive substances burn the body tissues and if swallowed may burn the mouth and the esophagus. More rarely, they may actually burn through the esophagus, causing a perforation requiring surgical treatment. Milk can help dilute and neutralize corrosives, especially if given at an early stage. Vomiting is not likely to be helpful in this case and may cause further damage (see Vomiting).

The ethylene glycol in antifreeze is converted by the body to oxalic acid, a substance that can damage the brain and kidneys. Some antifreezes also contain methyl alcohol, which the body converts into substances that damage the optic nerves and cause blindness. Other products, such as model aircraft fuel and rubbing alcohol, also contain methyl alcohol.

Acetaminophen, when taken in an overdose, leads to liver damage. At first there are no symptoms, but damage can be done to the cells in the liver because a small amount of the drug is converted into a poisonous substance. There are antidotes that can be very effective in preventing liver damage, provided they are given within 24 hours (see Liver and Liver Diseases). Aspirin can also be poisonous, but it has no known antidote. Of the many other poisons, each has its own toxic effect on the body, so that a doctor can often suspect a certain poison has been taken simply because of the signs or symptoms.

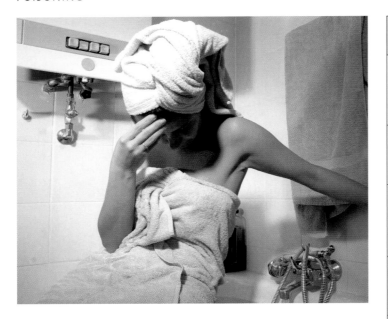

▲ *Dizziness and headaches due to carbon dioxide poisoning can result from gas leakage in a defective boiler heating system.*

Symptoms

Vomiting is one of the most important symptoms of poisoning; it is usually due to irritation or burning of the stomach but sometimes occurs because the poison has reached the part of the brain that controls the vomiting reflex. Convulsion is a symptom that can occur with some types of drugs for depression (see Convulsions). Other symptoms of poisoning include drowsiness, coma, and pain. Vomiting, drowsiness, and coma should always be taken seriously and help should be sought immediately. Some painkillers may cause no symptoms, but with most other poisons symptoms appear early if large doses are taken.

Treatment

In all cases of poisoning or suspected poisoning, the victim should be taken immediately to his or her local doctor or the emergency room of a hospital. This is also necessary when the victim has taken an overdose of tablets but there are no symptoms, since some medicines can have delayed effects. If possible, the patient should be accompanied and any tablets or household products that may have been taken should be brought along, with their containers.

It is sometimes possible and advisable to give immediate first-aid treatment in the home (see Emergencies). If a child has swallowed some pills and is conscious, it is sensible to attempt to induce vomiting by putting a finger down his or her throat. If this is not successful, do not persist; seek help at once. If the child has swallowed something believed to be corrosive, vomiting should not be induced, since this may cause further damage as the substance is regurgitated. Instead, the local emergency service should be called immediately.

Hospital treatment for any type of poisoning depends on the kind of poison and the amount that has been taken. Sometimes a drug called ipecac may be given to produce vomiting, or the stomach may be washed out with warm water passed through a tube (see Stomach Pump). All these measures prevent the poison from being absorbed further and reaching the bloodstream. Special techniques include giving lots of fluids so the poison is flushed out through the

kidneys; in very severe cases, the patient may be put on a dialysis (artificial kidney) machine. This treatment is normally used for aspirin poisoning. Dialysis machines are also able to remove certain drugs from the bloodstream (see Kidney Dialysis).

In a few cases, such as poisoning that is caused by taking iron tablets or certain types of painkilling drugs, antidotes can be given that bind with the poison or counteract its effects (see Iron). However, in most cases, only skilled nursing care and medical supervision are needed while the body overcomes the poison in its own way.

Outlook

Following treatment for poisoning, the patient usually does not suffer any aftereffects. Delayed reactions are rare, but if corrosives have been swallowed a doctor will examine the patient after a certain interval to see if the substance has had any side effect on the swallowing mechanism. A person who has taken poison when disturbed might attempt to do so again. Such people should be treated with great care and sympathy.

Preventing accidental poisoning

Bottles of cleaning fluids and bleach must never be left on the floor or stored at floor level in unlocked closets. The danger areas are: kitchen, bathroom, under the stairs, garage, and garden shed.

Closets containing dangerous substances must be locked or kept out of a child's reach. Medicines must always be kept in a locked closet and never left lying about in a room.

Never transfer any substance—whether it is poisonous or not—into an unlabeled container, particularly one such as a soft drink bottle or beer bottle. All household maintenance items, hobby items, and medicines should be clearly labeled.

Wash your hands immediately after handling any poisonous substance. Wash out used containers such as cans and buckets. Never leave them in the kitchen or near food.

Never keep unused drugs or medicines from an old prescription. Return them to your pharmacist, or if there are only a few tablets or drops of medicine left, flush them down the toilet.

Some medicines are packaged in the form of a pleasant-tasting syrup and many tablets also come in attractive colors and flavors. Never encourage children to take their tablets or medicines by pretending that you or they are taking sweets.

If you think someone has swallowed a poisonous substance, do not panic. By keeping a cool head and taking the right steps, you can still prevent serious damage. If in doubt, always consult your doctor or get to the hospital as soon as possible.

See also: Alcoholism; Aspirin and analgesics; Bites and stings; Coma; Environmental hazards; Food poisoning; Lung and lung diseases; Occupational hazards; Overdoses; Tranquilizers

Poliomyelitis

Since polio is so rare, is it still necessary to have my children vaccinated against it?

Yes, it is. The disease is close to eradication only because mass immunization has been successful. The virus does still exist, so it is important both for personal safety and in the interests of eradication for immunization to continue until the threat is past.

My husband had polio in the 1950s when he was a boy. Does this mean our children could be at risk?

So long as your children are vaccinated, there is no risk. Polio cannot be passed on through your husband and there is no risk of his carrying the virus now.

Can you get polio twice?

Since there are three different viruses that cause polio, it is theoretically possible to be infected three times; infection with one does not make you immune to the others. However, the chance that this will happen is extremely low. The polio vaccine gives lifelong immunity to all three types.

Does polio always cause paralysis?

No. Most people who become infected with the virus suffer only mild symptoms or none at all.

I have heard that polio is very infectious but can be caught only from those who have had paralysis as a symptom. Is this true?

No. Polio is infectious during the incubation period when the virus is multiplying. No one has nervous system symptoms at this time; these come after a few days but only in a small number of those infected. The most infectious time is when the symptoms are mild.

Poliomyelitis should be eradicated worldwide in the near future. Already, thanks to mass immunization programs, the Western Hemisphere is largely clear, and this once feared disease lingers only in southern Asia and Africa.

Poliomyelitis is a highly infectious disease caused by one of three related viruses. It affects the central nervous system and, depending on the severity and the virus involved, causes symptoms ranging from a mild flulike disorder to impaired breathing, muscle paralysis, and wasting.

Causes

Poliomyelitis, commonly called polio, is caused by a virus invading the motor cells of the spinal cord and parts of the brain (see Spinal Cord). The nerve cells involved are principally those that work the muscles of the limbs and those that control breathing and swallowing. The invasion of

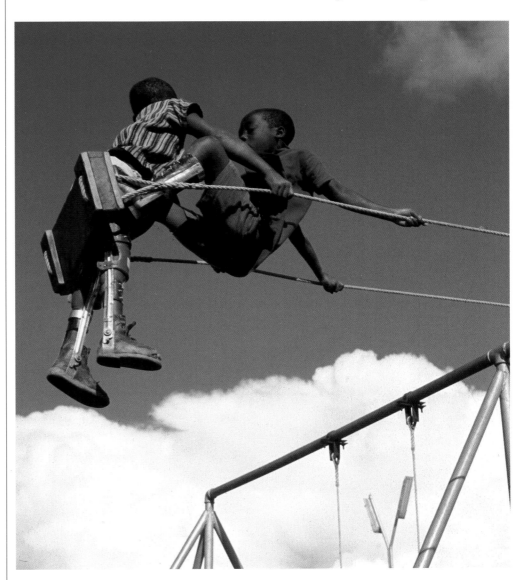

▲ *These African children are coping well with the effects of polio. Had they been vaccinated, of course, they would not have contracted this disabling disease.*

1633

these cells stimulates a reaction in the body's immune system; the nervous system becomes the field on which the battle is fought, and the resulting damage causes the disabling symptoms of the disease.

Symptoms

The disease starts with the polio virus multiplying in the lining of the throat and stomach. Often the infection stops here, causing what appears to be only a mild bout of gastroenteritis, or there may be no symptoms at all (see Gastroenteritis). In a few cases, symptoms indicating that the nervous system is involved may appear after a few days. Initially, these symptoms are mild muscle pains and aches. Again, in many people, the illness may have then run its course. If not, more serious signs, such as meningitis with neck stiffness and oversensitivity to light, may develop (see Meningitis). After this stage, or sometimes instead of it, a leg or an arm may become progressively weaker. In some cases this weakness may be extremely severe, affecting all the limbs and the muscles that control swallowing and breathing. This is probably the most

▼ *A woman receives physical therapy for a recurrence of polio, which she contracted 30 years previously.*

dangerous stage of polio because the patient may be unable to breathe without the aid of a respirator. If the brain stem—the part of the brain that controls the automatic functions of the body—is affected, the circulation may collapse, causing a drop in blood pressure and problems with the heart's rhythm.

Eventually, the acute inflammation that has been causing the symptoms settles down as the body's immune system fights the virus. The weakness and other symptoms may then fade to some extent as the undamaged nerve cells take over the function of those destroyed by the infection. However, any muscle wasting that has already occurred as a result of the loss of the muscle's nerve supply cannot be reversed.

Treatment and outlook

Viruses, unlike bacteria, are very difficult to get rid of once they have entered the body and started an infection. Antibiotics are not effective in destroying these germs. Therefore, once someone has contracted polio, treatment has to be restricted to trying to prevent the serious effects on the nervous system that cause irreparable damage.

Although there is no specific treatment for polio, there is much that can be done to treat aspects of the condition. The fever that

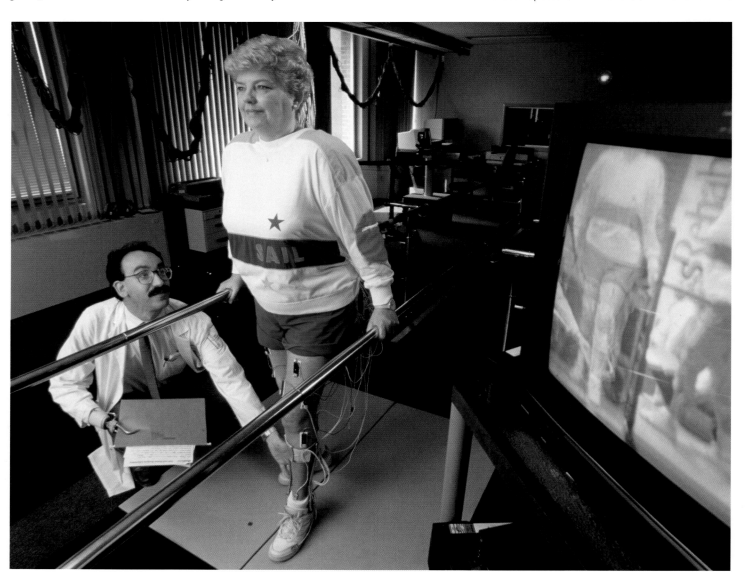

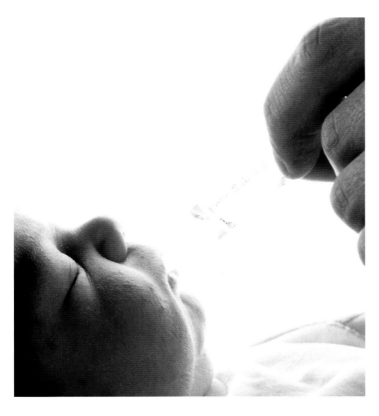

▲ *A baby receives the oral polio vaccination in liquid form.*

accompanies most of the symptoms of polio can be relieved by aspirin. If the nervous system is involved, the patient will be restricted to bed, since there is an increased risk of paralysis if the limbs are subjected to any exercise.

If the paralysis looks as if it is going to develop in the muscles concerned with swallowing or breathing, the patient's breathing power will be monitored. Should it then become necessary for a respirator to be used, a tracheostomy may be performed to make a small hole in the windpipe so that a breathing tube can be inserted (see Tracheostomy). The heart rhythm of the patient will also be kept under close observation.

Throughout the illness, if the patient's limbs are paralyzed, he or she must be nursed carefully to prevent bedsores. Physical therapy will also be given to maintain the suppleness of the affected limbs and to prevent the weakened muscles from wasting (see Physical Therapy). The vast majority of people who become infected with the polio virus do not get severe symptoms. However, they can pass on the virus to others in whom it may cause a far more serious illness.

Even when the nervous system has been attacked, the chances of recovery are good, although children and old people seem to do less well than young adults. Many polio victims do recover. They may be left with some wasting of muscles, but only a small number become disabled. Patients whose breathing is paralyzed usually recover enough to breathe on their own. Somebody who has had paralysis and then some recovery may suffer from post-polio syndrome, with pain and weakness in the recovered muscles.

Since polio is so difficult to treat once infection has occurred, it is vital that the virus is not allowed to take hold. Two factors have helped enormously in keeping infection at bay. One is the attention paid to sanitation in developed countries; as a result, the virus, which is shed

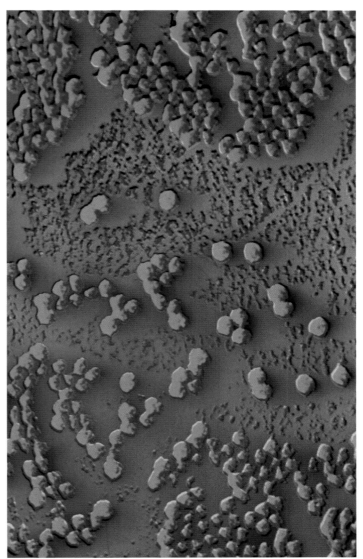

▲ *The polio virus—magnified here 20,000 times—is small and has a simple structure. However, in the days before vaccines it caused terrible epidemics.*

in feces, is less easily spread (see Feces). The second and more important factor is mass immunization. The international program began in 1988, when 35,000 cases were reported (see Public Health). By 1995, the number had fallen to 7,000 and the Western Hemisphere was free of polio. In 2002, there were 1,796 confirmed cases of polio from a total of nine countries, with India (1,509 cases), Nigeria (174 cases), and Bangladesh (90 cases) reporting the vast majority of cases. National immunization days, targeting all children under the age of five, continue in those countries at risk. The vaccination itself is simple. It is not administered by injection, but given in liquid form on a sugar lump. Most babies and children in the United States are vaccinated against polio and other diseases.

See also: **Hygiene; Immune system; Immunization; Infection and infectious diseases; Muscles; Nervous system; Paralysis; Vaccinations; Viruses**

Pollution

Questions and Answers

Is it true that aerosol hair sprays can damage the atmosphere?

Freon is a chlorofluorocarbon (CFC) compound that used to be present in aerosol sprays. Since 1978, the U.S. Environmental Protection Agency, the Food and Drug Administration, and the Consumer Products Safety Commission banned the use of chlorofluorocarbons as propellants in all nonessential aerosol products after they were found to damage the ozone layer. The only products that can contain CFCs are some medical products and commercial lubricants.

I am going to Britain on vacation, but I have heard that some British beaches are so polluted that it is dangerous to swim off them. Is this true?

Yes; recent surveys of Britain's beaches have shown that on some there is a risk from sewage pollution. The coastal Anti-Pollution League produces a "golden list" of clean beaches in England and Wales; check the list for any beaches you may be visiting.

If fluorine is a serious pollutant from industry, why is it added to drinking water?

Fluorine is beneficial in small quantities and harmful in large quantities. A small amount is present in plants and animals and this is essential for life. However, in some areas the water is deficient in fluorine and this deficiency has been linked to dental decay and poor tooth development in children. Small quantities added to water, often in the form of sodium fluoride, improve the structure of the teeth. Strangely, the first symptom of excess fluorine in the body is that the teeth become rough and mottled. Larger doses affect the bones and can be fatal.

Most of us are aware that smog and garbage dumps pollute the environment and affect our health. However, pollution also involves many dangerous, invisible substances present in the air, water, and soil.

"Pollution" is a broad term used to describe any change in the environment that affects the quality of human life. The causes vary, but they always involve some form of overproduction that leads to problems in the disposal of waste.

Although many people think that the concept of pollution was invented in the 1950s and 1960s, the detrimental effects it has on health have been recognized for centuries. For example, the ancient Greeks and Romans stored their garbage in designated areas outside the cities, but even this concentration of rotting waste led to epidemics of cholera, typhoid, and malaria (see Hygiene). By the Middle Ages the continuing increases in city populations contributed more to this type of pollution, and although city councils began to pass legislation against dumping garbage in canals, streams, and rivers, it had little effect (see Public Health).

However, the devastating effects of environmental pollution were not felt until the 19th century, when the Industrial Revolution created an explosive growth in industry. It happened first in Europe, then in North America, and later in Japan—the three areas of the world that even

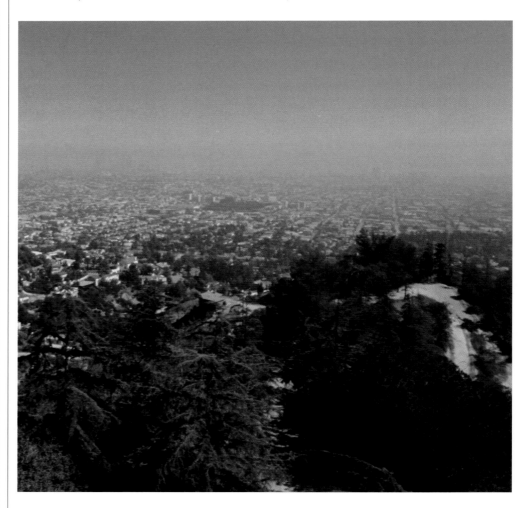

▲ *The infamous smog of Los Angeles is produced by the reaction of air pollutants with ultraviolet rays from sunlight.*

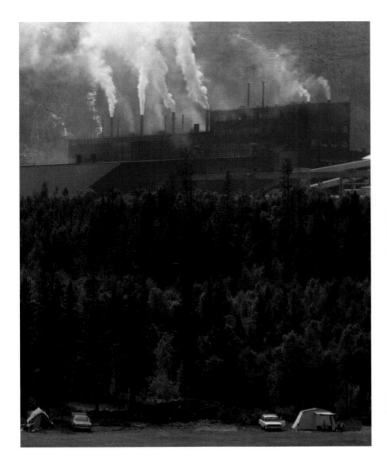

▲ *As industry spreads, there are fewer places where people can enjoy the open countryside.*

today are most affected by pollution, although pollution is now no longer a local problem but a global one.

It is convenient to divide pollution into three major categories: air, water, and soil. However, it is important to remember that each one affects the others.

Air pollution

Air pollution is caused by the discharge of by-products from the internal combustion engine, industrial processes, power stations, domestic consumption of fossil fuels (such as oil), and even the burning of agricultural waste. The actual substances that pollute the air are generally carbon monoxide, sulfur dioxide, nitrogen oxide, hydrocarbons, and particulate matter (dust and dirt).

Most people associate air pollution with the dramatic and deadly effects of smog. "Smog" is a contraction of the words "smoke" and "fog," and smog is indeed a mixture of smoke and fog combined with nitrogen oxide, hydrocarbons, and other pollutants.

The first federal clean-air act to control pollution was instigated in 1955 after a deadly smog enveloped the town of Donora, Pennsylvania. Twenty people were asphyxiated by the smog, which was caused by emissions from furnaces in the valley and town. The emissions contained sulfur dioxide, carbon monoxide, and metal dust. More than 7,000 people were hospitalized due to the effects of the smog. The subsequent investigation prompted legislation to control the pollution and efforts to assess and treat those whose health had been affected by the smog.

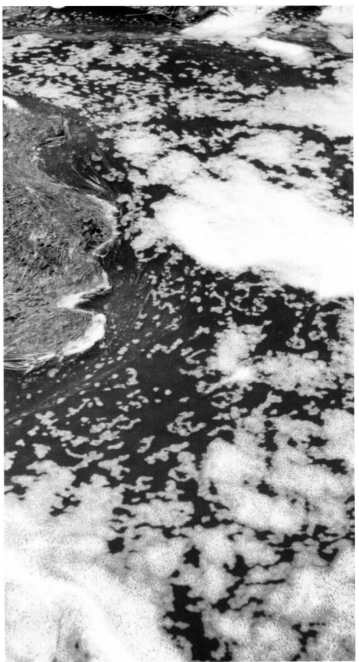

▲ *The discharge of detergents into rivers depletes the oxygen content of the water and is damaging to wildlife.*

The smog that afflicts cities in warm climates, such as Los Angeles, is a photochemical smog. It is caused by ultraviolet rays in sunshine reacting with the hydrocarbons and nitrogen oxides. Atmospheric stagnation occurs during temperature inversions; the air just above the cities is effectively sealed off and acute local air pollution results. The photochemical oxidants cause eye irritation and the nitrogen oxides cause other health problems, particularly in children; for example, children's susceptibility to influenza and other viral infections may be increased (see Influenza; Viruses).

Carbon monoxide from automobile exhausts displaces the oxygen in the body when it is inhaled (see Oxygen). At the

Questions and Answers

I've been told that where there is a large oil slick, the detergents that are used to disperse it cause more damage than the oil. Is this true?

Yes. Although the oil has a disastrous effect on the seabirds, it is a natural mixture of hydrocarbons that will be broken down eventually in the sea. The detergents are usually synthetic organic compounds and can persist for a long time.

When I spend a day shopping in New York City, I often feel dizzy. Is this dizziness due to a lack of oxygen in the air?

Almost certainly not. It may seem surprising, but the amount of oxygen is nearly the same in polluted air as in fresh air. There is probably less oxygen on top of the highest mountains than there is in a crowded city store. However, there is an increase in carbon monoxide where there is heavy traffic and this can dull the senses a little. Also, the number of people on subway trains and in the stores can cause the stuffiness that can make you feel dizzy, and high temperatures do not help.

Can city air polluted with gasoline fumes cause brain damage?

Yes; there is clear evidence that the lead in gasoline can cause brain damage. Governments take the threat seriously, and the amount of lead that is added to gasoline has now been reduced. Most cars now run on lead-free gasoline.

Is it true that living in a city is equivalent to smoking a pack of cigarettes a day in the country?

The two are not comparable. The risks of cigarette smoking are specific and well known and greatly exceed the risks to nonsmokers who live in cities. Moreover, although urban life does involve exposure to more pollution than rural life, the degree—and to some extent the type—of pollution varies from city to city.

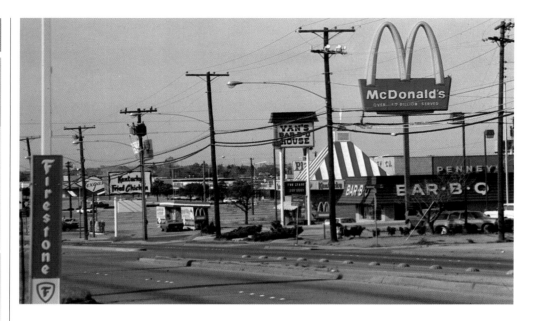

▲ *When towns spill out into rural areas, the natural environment is often eclipsed by one that is totally artificial.*

concentrations often found in the air in large cities, it can cause a slowing of the reflexes and a dulling of the senses. These effects can lead to an increase in the number of automobile accidents, since people are not as alert as usual.

Sulfur dioxide is released into the atmosphere when coal and oil are burned, and it can often be detected in heavy industrial areas by a sharp, acrid smell in the air. As it reaches the air, the sulfur dioxide mixes with the moisture that is present and turns into sulfuric acid. This then returns to earth in a liquid form called acid rain.

Acid rain is a serious form of pollution. It causes inconvenience by tarnishing polished copper and brass door fittings and attacking statues and buildings, but it can also have a devastating effect on people and wildlife. Sulfur compounds can cause permanent damage to the respiratory system

▼ *"Dead Fjord," Sweden, where chemicals from a local factory polluted the water.*

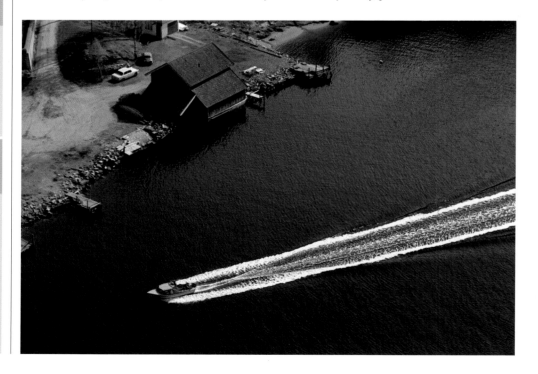

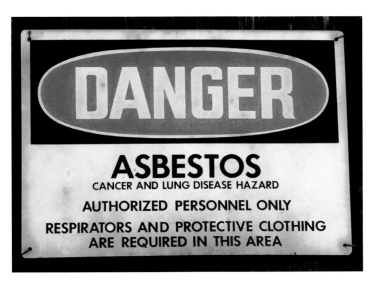

▲ *The mineral asbestos has been used in commercial products since the late 19th century, owing to its resistance to heat and fire. However, it was found to cause a potentially fatal disease called asbestosis, in which people exposed to asbestos could suffer scarring of the lungs, breathing problems, heart failure, and cancer. Since the 1970s, regulations have been introduced limiting the use of asbestos in many products.*

by affecting lung tissue and the bronchi (air passages in the lungs), and these compounds have an irritant effect on the eyes, causing them to tear.

Acid rain decreases the forest yields in Scandinavia and parts of North America, and it has caused the elimination of fish in many lakes. The sulfur pollutants that fall on Norway and Sweden do not even arise in those countries, but originate from the industrial centers of Great Britain and Germany.

Ozone is released into the atmosphere by electrical equipment and can also be generated on hot sunny days. Although ozone is widely believed to aggravate respiratory conditions, such as asthma and emphysema, the supporting evidence is inconclusive (see Pulmonary Disorders).

Fluorine is particularly associated with the smoke from the chimneys of brickyards. The problem with fluorine is that once it is deposited, it is not broken down. It therefore concentrates in the soil, and the plants concentrate it further. However, fluorine is a rare pollutant, and the potential damage that it can inflict is better known than actual cases of fluorine poisoning (see Fluoride).

"Particulate pollution" is a rather general term; it covers all the dust and dirt in the atmosphere. Naturally, this kind of pollution causes more problems on and around industrial sites and in cities. The effects of these dust particles on health appear to be twofold.

First, the incidence of lung cancer is higher in cities than in the country, and this difference is thought to be directly attributable to the amount of dirt in the atmosphere. Second, diseases of the respiratory tract, such as asthma, bronchitis, and emphysema, are most common in cities (see Lung and Lung Diseases).

Water pollution

Unlike air pollution, water pollution is a visible catastrophe. The well-publicized oil slicks that ruin beaches and kill so many seabirds are evidence of water pollution, as are the unsightly collections of domestic garbage that are found on our beaches.

For a long time, the earth's oceans were the one natural system that could absorb the waste produced by humankind and break it down before it became dangerous. This is no longer the case. Industrial and domestic wastes have reached such a level that the seas and oceans are beginning to reach their capacity for breaking down the excess chemicals produced. The Mediterranean Sea is a classic example of a sea that has become so polluted that in many areas it is devoid of animal and plant life and is unsafe for swimming.

Pollutants that reach the sea generally originate inland and are carried down by rivers. Pollution of rivers was one of the earliest environmental problems to be recognized. Water pollutants are made up of both organic and inorganic material. Organic pollutants include sewage, synthetic detergents, and a wide range of pesticides.

Although much sewage is treated before it is discharged into seas or rivers, a surprising amount is not. A great many beaches are contaminated by raw sewage, and feces and contraceptives floating in the water are not uncommon in some areas. Excess sewage has the effect of reducing the oxygen content of water and thus killing wildlife; it also carries bacterial and viral diseases as well as parasitic organisms (see Bacteria; Parasites; Viruses).

Detergents and pesticides

Detergents are everyday and, some might say, essential commodities. The most ancient is soap; this is broken down during sewage treatment and causes very little harm. However, after World War I, synthetic chemicals were developed that do not break down easily.

When these detergents are discharged into rivers, persistent quantities of thick foam build up into vast banks. These detergent

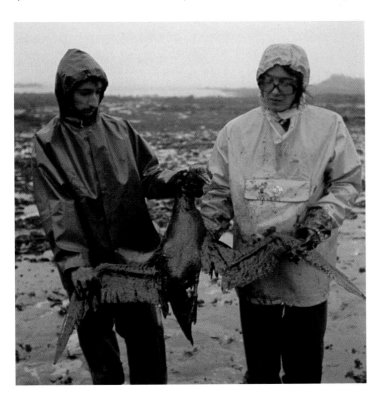

▲ *Beaches are threatened by oil spills, often with drastic results for wildlife.*

▶ *After soil at this site was severely contaminated with pollutants in 1977, it was removed and disinfected.*

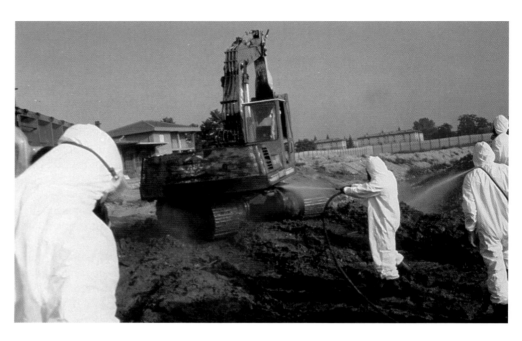

banks usually occur away from the sewage outfall and exist in places where the water has already begun to clear. This is because dirty water produces little foam, as can be seen when a person washes his or her hair when it is very dirty and the shampoo does not lather up well. Detergents can not only be harmful to people but also cause death to many species of wildlife by reducing the oxygen content of the water.

Pesticides find their way into the rivers from agricultural land and can cause a great deal of damage to both people and wildlife. Organochloride pesticides, like DDT, were concentrated as they passed through the food chain, and these pollutants have caused death in many species of fish and seabirds. They also caused a reduction in wildlife populations by interfering with the breeding cycles of some species. Circulation of DDT once occurred throughout the world, but in many countries its use is now banned.

The inorganic pollutants fall into two categories: fertilizers and industrial waste. They usually contain heavy metals, such as lead or mercury. Because of the increased use of inorganic fertilizers by agriculturalists, large quantities of these fertilizers are being leached from the land and washed into streams, rivers, and lakes. There, they stimulate the growth of aquatic plants, and as a result many waterways become oxygen-poor swamps.

Mercury contamination

Industrial waste that carries metals into the water can cause serious illnesses. Mercury poisoning is probably one of the most dramatic and best-known of these.

In the 1950s worldwide concern arose when it was found that fishermen, their families and pets, and the local seabirds near Minimata Bay in Japan were suffering from an unexplained disease. The victims suffered from muscle weakness, blindness, and brain damage, and in extreme cases coma, paralysis, and death resulted. Since the villagers ate mainly fish, the fish were analyzed and shown to contain high concentrations of mercury compounds, which were eventually traced to the waste discharged from a local factory.

Throughout the next two decades there were numerous other scares about mercury poisoning associated with contaminated fish, particularly in Canada, the United States, and Scandinavia, and laws were passed to limit the amount of mercury waste discharged into rivers, lakes, and seas. Most of this came from mercury used in the chemical industry and other industries, such as paint manufacturing.

The natural balance of many rivers and some parts of the coastline is altered by industry—particularly by power stations—because the temperature of the water is raised. Although warm water itself is not damaging, it can increase the effects of organic pollution and can change the natural flora and fauna of the river. No doubt this heat pollution will increase in the future and needs to be carefully watched and monitored.

Soil pollution

Soil pollution causes less concern than air and water pollution simply because soil is not mobile, and pollution therefore tends to be localized. Soil pollution occurs from persistent pesticides that remain for years in slag heaps from mines, and in industrial areas where over the years many tons of dust and dirt have been deposited from factory chimneys.

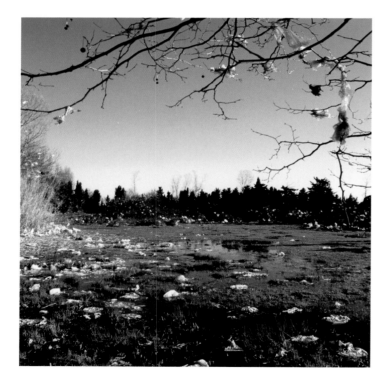

▲ *The litter strewn over this swamp causes health risks to the local wildlife. Birds and other swamp inhabitants may choke on the litter or get caught up in it.*

Soil pollution does not usually cause a severe health hazard, since in heavily polluted areas no crops are grown and so the chemicals cannot be passed on to people. A danger does exist, though, when plants concentrate residues from the soil and increase their concentration above certain recognized safe levels.

Other forms of pollution

There are some types of pollution that do not fit conveniently into any of the above three categories, but like air, water, and soil pollution, they are all created by humankind.

Noise pollution can be defined as unwanted sound and is a growing problem that is affecting our environment. The noise generated by industry, automobiles, and airplanes is not merely an inconvenience, but a serious health hazard. Pulse and respiratory rates can be increased by sound, and persistent noise can cause ulcers and hypertension. It has even been suggested that noise can cause heart attacks in people with a weak or otherwise damaged heart.

There are also types of pollution which do no physical harm to people or animals, but which can be aesthetically annoying. Billboards and flashing neon signs, power lines, and ugly buildings can all be classed as visual pollutants.

Pollution by light has also been of great concern to astronomers, if not anyone else, because the glare from streetlights and domestic lights around the world affects detailed observation of the stars and planets. This light pollution results because the light rays that are emitted 24 hours a day from the world's cities are scattered by particles in the polluted air to create a type of blanket over the earth. To avoid this problem, most large-scale astronomical observatories have now been built on, or moved to, remote or very

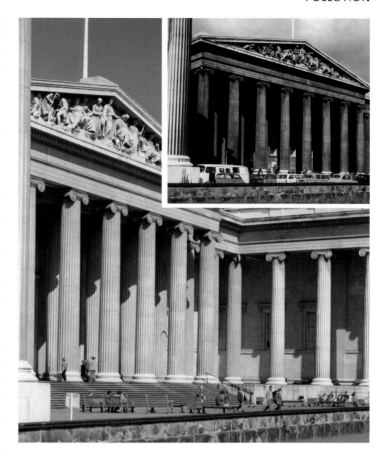

▲ *Cleaning buildings in London, such as the British Museum, removes decades of grime (inset) that also pollutes the air.*

high locations, such as the South Pole or mountains in places such as Hawaii, New Mexico, and Arizona.

Radiation poisoning

Radiation levels in the environment have been declining since the 1960s after international agreements to stop the testing of atomic bombs in the atmosphere, under water, and in space. However, man-made radiation still comes from medical X rays and electronic devices such as television sets (see X Rays). Medical use accounts for more than 90 percent of the radiation that an individual will be exposed to in his or her lifetime.

Serious damage caused by radiation has usuallly been restricted to people who have lived close to atomic testing sites, or who are exposed to it during their work. However, after the meltdown of the nuclear reactor at Chernobyl, Ukraine, in 1986, a number of people died of radiation poisoning immediately. The long-term effects of lower-level exposures from this disaster are still unknown. With the proliferation of nuclear waste and the problems of its storage, this waste could have serious effects in the future. High doses can cause cancers, such as leukemia, and constant low-level radiation causes genetic damage (see Cancer; Leukemia).

See also: Acid rain; Air pollution; Asbestosis; Environmental hazards; Lead poisoning; Noise; Occupational hazards; Ozone layer; Poisoning; Radiation sickness

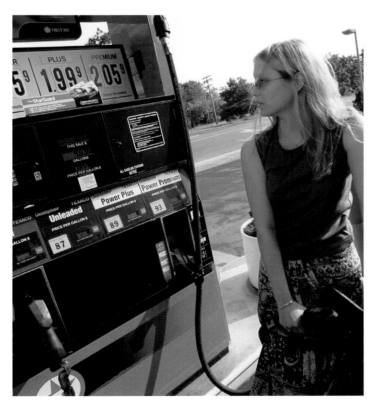

▲ *Most cars now run on lead-free gas, thus reducing the amount of lead pollution, which can cause brain damage.*

Polyps

I have a polyp in my colon. Will I need to have it removed?

Yes, because there is a slight chance that it may turn malignant later on. However, in most cases polyps in the colon can be removed by endoscopic surgery via the anus that involves no incision and only moderate discomfort.

Are some people more prone to polyps than others?

Yes. There is a condition that runs in families in which the entire colon becomes filled with polyps. They appear early in adult life and cause symptoms such as bleeding. The colon usually has to be removed because of the risk that cancer will develop in later life. When this condition is found, other family members should also be checked to see if they are similarly affected. If the same condition is found, they will also need surgery.

Can a polyp regrow or appear elsewhere in the body after it has been removed?

Yes. For example, nasal polyps tend to regrow, especially if nasal decongestant sprays are overused, or if the person suffers from hay fever. There may also be an increased incidence of polyps in the intestines if a person has already had one removed. However, these polyps may not be regrowths of the same polyp, but new polyps arising from the lining membrane.

If I have a polyp in my womb, should I avoid getting pregnant until it has been removed?

Ask your gynecologist for advice. A small polyp would not cause any harm, but a large one, or a group of polyps, might do so, because they can become compressed and suddenly degenerate, causing a slight risk of miscarriage.

Any small growths that are attached to a stalk and arise from a mucous membrane lining are called polyps. They always need medical attention, but they are easily identified and treated.

Most polyps are due to an overgrowth of the mucous membrane lining at a particular site so that a small lump is formed (see Membranes; Mucus). They may occur singly or in large numbers and may be present from birth or develop later in life. Common sites of polyps are the nose, larynx, stomach, intestines, and uterus. Most polyps are benign, some are potentially malignant, and a few are malignant from the start of their growth (see Malignancy).

Nasal polyps

Nasal polyps are attached to the mucous membrane lining the nose, and consist of swellings that can grow as big as a grape if left untreated. They occur in people who have frequent colds and hay fever, and are also a cause of nasal infections (see Common Cold; Hay Fever). Equally, they can cause infections in the sinuses, the cavities in the bones of the face, by blocking the tiny communicating channels between the nasal cavity and the sinuses.

Nasal polyps can cause one side of the nose to become blocked, or excessive discharge to come from the nose for a long time. The polyps can be seen with the help of a special viewing speculum. They are easily removed under general anesthesia by passing a wire loop around each one in turn and snaring it. This is a relatively minor procedure, although further treatment may be needed at a later date if more polyps develop.

POLYPS IN THE UTERUS

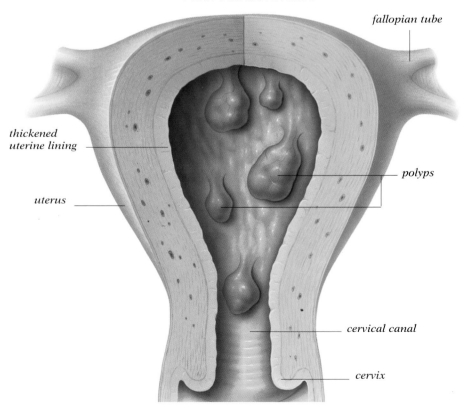

▲ *Endometrial polyps grow out from the mucous lining of the uterus. Although usually benign, they can cause menstrual irregularities, but they can be treated.*

Polyps in the intestines

Polyps in the intestines occur most often in the large intestine and rectum, but are sometimes found in the small intestine, especially in certain rare congenital syndromes. In the large intestine, polyps may be single or multiple, very small or as large as 1.2 inches (3 cm) in diameter.

In the condition called familial polyposis coli, hundreds of small polyps develop in the colon. Several members of a family may be affected in this way. Because of the high risk that one or more of these polyps may turn malignant, the colon is always removed and the small intestine is joined to the rectum (see Colon and Colitis).

However, most cases of polyps in the large intestine are not hereditary and usually appear in the lower part of the colon. A person with intestinal polyps may notice blood or excessive mucus in the feces, and lower abdominal pain as the intestine attempts to pass the polyp along as if it were feces. This pulls on the polyp and the intestine wall, causing pain.

Polyps in the intestines can be seen with the aid of a sigmoidoscope (a hollow tube passed into the rectum) or a colonoscope, which is a long flexible viewing instrument that can be maneuvered through the bends of the colon (see Endoscopy). A

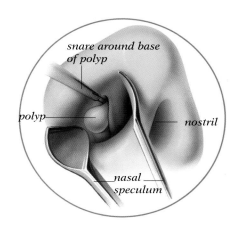

▲ *Nasal polyps are removed painlessly under anesthesia. A wire loop, or snare, is passed over each one, pulled tight at the base, and the polyp gently eased away.*

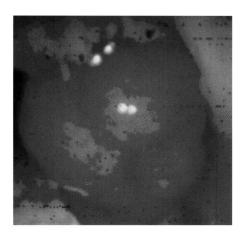

▲ *This polyp, 1.2 in. (3 cm) in size, was taken from the colon of a patient. It was removed in minutes by a colonoscope, thus avoiding the need for abdominal surgery.*

barium enema, in which the intestine shows up on an X ray, may also be used to clarify the diagnosis (see Barium Liquids; Enema; X Rays).

Polyps must always be removed because of the symptoms they cause and because they are likely to turn malignant if they grow larger than 0.4 inch (about 1 cm) in diameter. A polyp can be removed with a colonoscope. When a polyp is removed with a colonoscope, the patient is given intravenous (IV) sedation before the instrument is passed into the rectum. The polyp is identified and a long wire with a loop at the end is threaded through the colonoscope. The loop is put over the polyp and is pulled tight, and an electric current is passed through the wire. This cauterizes the base of the polyp so that it can be removed without bleeding. The procedure is usually done on an outpatient basis.

Polyps in the uterus

Polyps may arise in the uterus either from the mucous membrane lining the inside of the uterus or from the cervix (the neck of the womb). They may become apparent in the patient because of heavy periods or because of bleeding between periods or after menopause (see Menopause).

These polyps are normally removed by the procedure of dilatation and curettage, or D & C. In this operation, the lining of the uterus is scraped out, together with any polyps that are present. Sometimes polyps in the uterus are an indication of fibroids, which are fibrous swellings in the muscular wall of the uterus.

In cases such as these, it may be necessary to remove the uterus to cure the symptoms (see Hysterectomy) .

NASAL POLYPS AND THEIR REMOVAL

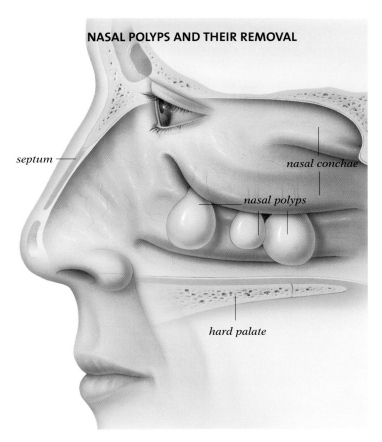

septum
nasal conchae
nasal polyps
hard palate

▲ *Nasal polyps are soft, round swellings that may occur singly or in large numbers. They often arise within the sinus cavities as well as in the nasal cavity.*

Outlook

Polyps are easily dealt with by using modern surgical techniques. A patient who has had one or more polyps removed will continue to be monitored for some time in case of any possible recurrence of the problem.

> See also: **Cervix and cervical smears; Colonoscopy; Dilatation and curettage; Fibroids; Growths; Larynx and laryngitis; Menstruation; Nose; Sigmoidoscopy; Stomach; Uterus**

Postoperative care

The effects of surgery extend far beyond the operation itself. How quickly and successfully a patient recovers depends enormously on the postoperative (after surgery) care he or she receives.

Questions and Answers

When I visited my friend after she had surgery, I thought she looked awful. Why is the body so weak and frail after a major operation?

There are many reasons. First of all, major surgery causes severe trauma to the body. The body reacts to this in certain ways, by concentrating on healing the area of the surgery and switching resources from maintaining the rest of the body, which leads to a generalized weakening. Second, a major operation affects the body's immune mechanisms so that it is more susceptible to infections. Third, it is possible that the anesthesia used has an effect that is not yet understood. Fourth, medication to relieve pain can make the patient feel very weak.

Why do some people take longer than others to recover from the same surgery?

This depends on many physical, psychological, and social factors. For example, undernourishment or the presence of other diseases before surgery may delay healing afterward. The willpower of the patient is a big factor in recovery time; some people can get going much faster than others. Social factors also play a part; some patients get a lot of help and support from friends or family.

If further surgery is needed, how soon after the first operation can this be done?

There are certain rules for this. The surgeon will not subject the patient to a second operation immediately after the first unless it is strictly necessary. It is usually better to allow the patient to recover for several weeks and become stronger. Reoperating on the same site a week after the first surgery is difficult technically because of the acute healing processes that are going on.

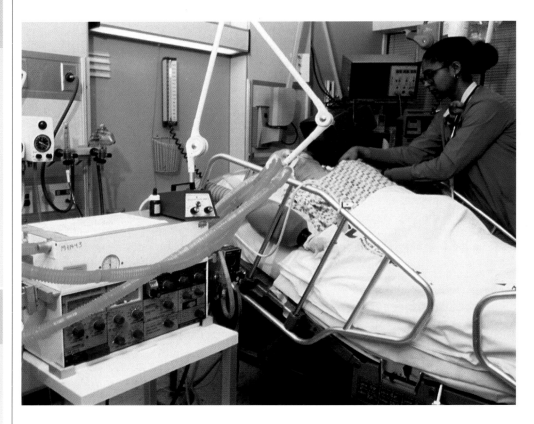

▲ *After major surgery, it may be necessary for the patient to be treated in an intensive care unit rather than on an ordinary ward.*

Postoperative care involves several aspects concerned with the recovery of the patient, beginning with the care of the patient immediately after surgery has taken place, and ending with his or her complete recovery.

The progress of recovery depends on several factors: the type of surgery involved, the patient's awareness of the various stages that occur after surgery, the patient's general state of health, and the facilities available at the hospital for postoperative care.

The recovery room

After surgery, the patient is taken immediately from the operating room to the recovery room, where specially trained nurses will monitor the patient's postoperative progress for a short while. The recovery room has the advantage of having specialized equipment such as oxygen sets and blood pressure measuring equipment more readily at hand than on the other hospital floors.

The nurse in the recovery room will carefully monitor the patient's blood pressure and pulse, consciousness level, and airway. An unconscious patient will have no cough reflex, and if secretions accumulate at the back of the throat, they can be sucked down the trachea (windpipe) and end up in the lungs where serious damage leading to pneumonia could occur (see Pneumonia). By positioning the patient carefully, the nurse is able to ensure that a clear airway is maintained at all times, and that there is no danger of the patient's tongue falling backward and causing choking.

If there is any increase in the amount of fluid at the back of the throat, the nurse will use suction equipment to clear the airway. Excessive fluid in the airway could occur, for example, after surgery on the nose or the mouth itself, or after the tonsils have been removed (see Tonsils). As the patients regain consciousness, however, they will be able to protect their own airway by coughing out any inhaled secretions.

As well as monitoring blood pressure, pulse, and respiration, the nurse also notes any change at the site of the surgery, and monitors any drainage from tubes that may have been inserted during surgery. Patients who have had their prostate gland removed, for example, have a tube in the bladder, and fluid is run in through this tube and out again to prevent blood clots in the bladder and blockage of the tube (see Prostate Gland). The recovery nurse will ensure that the tube remains in the correct position and that continual drainage occurs. Finally, when the nurses are satisfied that the patient is fully conscious and can be moved safely, the patient is then taken on a gurney back to his or her room.

Nursing care

In some hospitals, the patient's own bed can be brought down to the operating room and he or she can be transferred to it.

▼ *The patient is taken to the recovery room immediately after surgery, while still unconscious.*

Back on the floor, the same nursing observations are continued, but at less frequent intervals. At this stage, as the effect of the anesthetic wears off, the patient may begin to experience pain from the surgery. Anesthetists will, however, usually anticipate pain and order an appropriate painkilling injection.

Signs that a patient is developing pain include restlessness, sweating, and an increase in pulse rate, apart from the obvious effect of pain on a patient's well-being. An injection is usually given at this stage; its effects may last several hours (see Injections).

It should be emphasized, however, that some patients experience very little pain after surgery, and need no painkilling injections at all (see Pain).

From the patient's point of view, waking up after an anesthetic can be a pleasant or unpleasant experience. An anesthetic will have different effects on different people. For the majority, it is like waking up from a deep sleep; for others there may be unpleasant side effects. Nausea is one such side effect, although actual vomiting can usually be prevented by giving special injections (see Nausea). Some patients feel very confused and disoriented for a while, and others experience peculiar sensations in the body, such as tingling. These effects are usually very short-lived.

All patients vary considerably in the length of time that they are affected by the anesthetic. Some patients will really wake up only several hours after coming back to the floor, whereas others will be fully awake by the time they reach the floor.

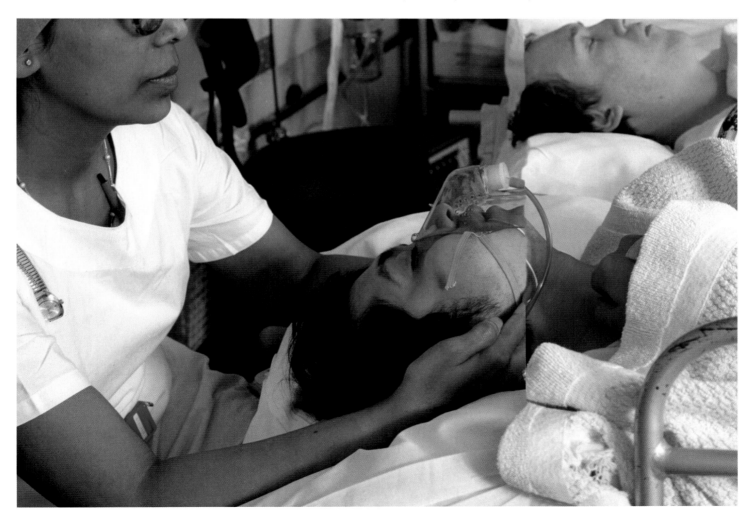

I'm going into the hospital soon for surgery. Can you give me an idea of how long the wound will be painful?

This depends very much on the site and size of the wound. Some wounds are much more painful than others. As a general rule, though, the pain should be much less after two days, and painkilling injections should no longer be required. Usually after a week there is virtually no pain at all.

Can surgery actually cause the body to go into a state of shock, thereby complicating the issue?

Yes. When doctors use the term "shock," they are referring to any condition in which the body's blood circulation is impaired to such a degree that the body tissues are not being supplied with enough oxygen. This can happen if the patient loses a lot of blood during surgery and it is not replaced, or if the surgery disturbs an infected area, such as an abscess, and leads to an infection in the blood.

The doctors told my father to rest after his surgery, but he finds it hard to sit still. Can he do himself harm by ignoring this advice?

He will probably not do himself any harm, but he may exhaust himself, and therefore find that he has set his recovery back somewhat. In the first few weeks after surgery, the body is putting all its energies into healing itself, and there is very little energy left for other physical activities.

My wife has just had surgery on the stomach and is being fed with an intravenous tube. Why?

After any surgery on the abdomen, the intestines stop working for a short time. Your wife cannot eat or drink during this time, and so instead fluid is fed into a vein. Once her intestines have started working again, however, she will be able to eat and drink normally.

Intensive care

Some surgery, especially major heart surgery, involves the use of so much specialized monitoring equipment after the operation that it would be impossible for the patient to be nursed on an ordinary floor. Instead, special facilities have been developed to deal with every need of such patients. These are called intensive care units.

As well as containing special equipment for monitoring patients, intensive care units also contain mechanical respirators that take over the movements of breathing and are connected up to the patient via a tube in the trachea (see Respirators).

The effects of surgery

The day after surgery, the effects of the anesthetic should begin to wear off completely, and the patient will be left with the normal postoperative problems that are associated with the surgical wound itself.

One of the main effects of having a wound is that the patient becomes relatively immobile, and it is this immobility that both nurses and patient must counter almost immediately.

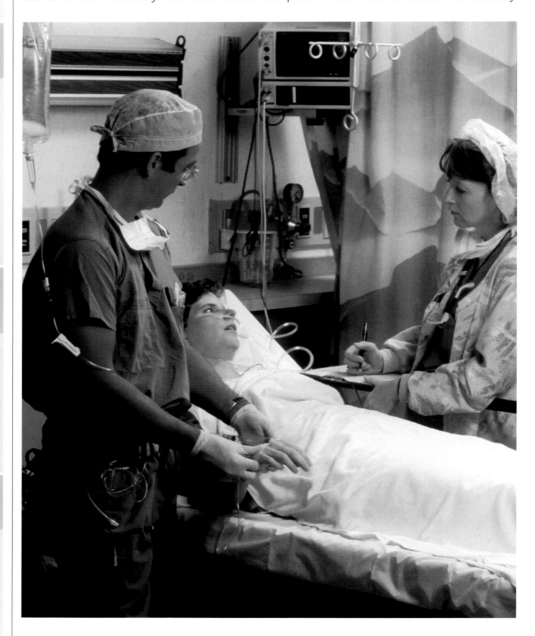

▲ *As a woman wakes from surgery in the recovery room, the anesthesiologist checks her condition. Specialized nurses will keep a constant check on her progress.*

However, because any movement may cause pain, the patient is obviously more inclined to lie as still as possible. It is here that a little gentle coaxing by a sympathetic nursing staff is needed. The ability of a patient to become mobile quickly after surgery can make all the difference between an uncomplicated recovery from surgery and one that is marred by thrombosis in the leg veins (see Thrombosis), or by chest infection. Basically, movement increases the circulation of blood, and oxygen, around the body and thus aids recovery.

Surgical wounds are sutured with very strong materials, and it would be virtually impossible to burst the stitches by too much activity (see Sutures). Most patients are mobile the day after surgery, and if the operation was a minor one they are encouraged to walk about. It has been shown that the incidence of complications is much lower in patients who are mobilie soon after surgery. The pain of surgery becomes less severe very quickly afterward, and any residual pain can be relieved with injections or tablets (see Painkillers).

What to tell the patient

Anybody waking up after surgery is going to be curious about how the operation went. More often than not, of course, the surgeon is able to tell him or her that the surgery proceeded smoothly.

In some cases, however, particularly where cancer is suspected, people often vary in how much they wish to be told (see Cancer). Some people want to know everything about the details of their surgery, while others could not care less, as long as they feel they are getting better.

Doctors often find out before surgery how much the patient wants to know, and it is usually fairly obvious into which category the patient falls. Most doctors are prepared to tell the patient everything if the patient asks, but may not force such details on the patient if he or she does not ask for them to be explained.

Visitors

Obviously, a patient's close relatives will want to come and visit as soon as the patient is out of surgery. However, it must be remembered that, for the patient, a visit can be a very tiring experience so soon after an operation. The all too familiar scene is of a hospital room with six visitors sitting around the bed all talking to each other and of an exhausted patient lying in the middle of it. The sensible hospital nurse will try to prevent this and, for everyone's sake, will usually impose some sort of restriction on the number of visitors allowed at any one time.

At home

The length of time a patient must stay in the hospital after surgery before being allowed home depends on the type of surgery undertaken and the conditions at home. A young, fit girl living with her family would obviously be able to manage much better than an old woman living on her own, even though they both may have had the same surgery.

When a patient is allowed to go home after surgery, he or she usually feels very weak for at least a few weeks (see Fatigue). Postoperative exercise may have been limited to very short walks in the hospital. It is only when the patient gets home that postoperative weakness really kicks in. For example, patients who have had major surgery, such as the removal of a lung or the colon, often find that it can be as much as three months before they feel

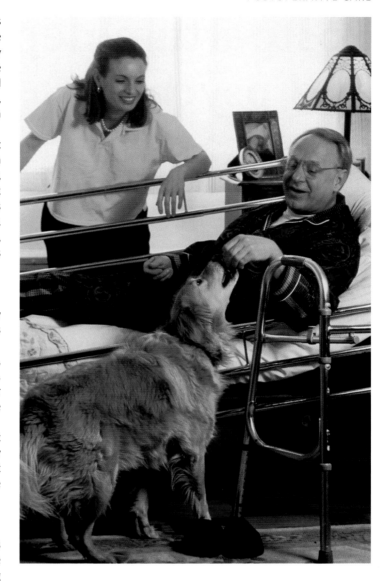

▲ *Postoperative care does not end when the patient leaves the hospital. He or she may be too weak to do anything at home for a while. However, a strong support network of family and friends can promote a speedy recovery back to normal health.*

well again. During this time, the patient will have to visit the surgeon's office for ongoing assessment of his or her progress. During these visits any queries a patient may have about the surgery or new concerns arising from the recovery stages can be answered by the doctor.

There are many things that can help a speedy recovery from surgery, and these include both physical and mental factors. Obviously, the will to recover will vary from person to person, although other factors, such as the overall health of the patient, are also important to recovery.

However, most modern hospitals are now very well equipped to anticipate and deal with a wide range of postoperative scenarios.

> *See also:* Anesthetics; Blood pressure; Healing; Hospitals; Intensive care unit; Operating room; Oxygen; Pulse; Surgery; Unconsciousness

Postpartum depression and psychosis

Postpartum depression (PPD) and psychosis is a condition embracing a number of physical and emotional changes that a woman can experience after giving birth to a baby. The condition can be treated with medication, counseling, and support from family and friends.

Having a baby can be one of the most joyful events in a woman's life. However, it can also be difficult and stressful at times because of major changes in lifestyle and the considerable demands of motherhood.

Any depression that a woman suffers after childbirth can be exacerbated if she does not have emotional support or if she is having to contend with other stressful life events. It may be hard

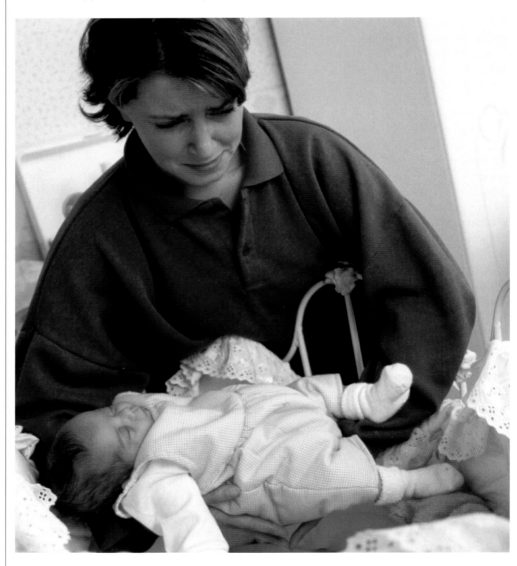

▲ *Women with PPD find it hard to confront the daily care and attention that a baby requires. Without adequate support, they may find the stress of trying to cope unbearable.*

for some women to admit that they have negative feelings during what is generally expected to be a particuary happy time in their lives (see Birth).

In fact, the period following childbirth poses a substantial risk to the mental health of women. The risk in the year following the delivery of a child is greater than the risk at any other time of a woman's life—at least 10 percent of women suffer a definite depressive illness during this year and up to 30 percent have some degree of depression. Approximately four in 1,000 women need hospital admission for depression, and two per 1,000 are admitted with a diagnosis of psychosis. In 80 percent of these cases it will be the woman's first episode of a psychotic illness. In contrast, during pregnancy a woman's mental health tends to be excellent, and pregnant women are much less likely to require psychiatric care, or to take an overdose or to commit suicide in any other way.

Baby blues

It is both common and natural for a new mother to experience mood swings after the birth. She may feel elated one minute, then sad and tearful the next. The extreme physical and emotional changes of having a baby can result in a woman's feeling sad, anxious, and afraid (see Anxiety). These feelings usually pass quickly and are often referred to as the "baby blues." Baby blues can last for as little as a few hours or up to two weeks after delivery.

About eight in 10 women are affected by baby blues after childbirth, and about one woman in 1,000 goes on to develop a severe psychiatric condition called postpartum psychosis. However, if these mild feelings do not go away or if they get worse, a woman may be suffering from postpartum depression (PPD). PPD is a serious, but temporary, illness that requires urgent treatment. It usually occurs from a few days after birth to six months later. PPD can happen after any birth, not just after that of a first child.

Warning signs

The symptoms of postpartum depression can prevent a new mother from being able to do the things she needs to do on a daily basis. The common warning signs of PPD include feeling sad, depressed, inadequate, or irritable; crying a lot; losing energy and interest in life; feeling tired and having problems sleeping; experiencing an unexplained weight loss or gain; and having trouble concentrating and making decisions. Sometimes a mother suffering from PPD worries about harming herself or her baby, or has no interest in her baby.

It is important for a woman to seek immediate help from a health care professional if she thinks she is affected by this condition. If she does not get treatment quickly, symptoms can worsen and last for as long as a year. The experiences of women who have PPD vary greatly, and some of the symptoms, such as sleep problems, weight fluctuations, and fatigue, are normal following childbirth (see Fatigue; Sleep and Sleep Problems; Weight). However, one of the symptoms of PPD must be either depression or a considerably reduced interest in nearly all activities.

Causes of PPD

PPD is like any other form of depression. All that distinguishes it is that it happens around the time of childbirth. No one knows exactly what causes PPD, but hormones are increasingly believed to trigger its symptoms. The female hormones estrogen and progesterone increase greatly during pregnancy (see Estrogen). In the first 24 hours after

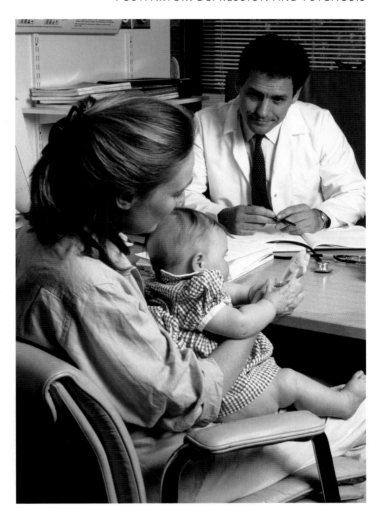

▲ *A woman with symptoms of PPD should not hesitate to see her doctor, who will diagnose her condition and prescribe the appropriate medical treatment if she does have PPD.*

delivery, the levels of these hormones drop drastically and continue to drop to the levels they were at before the woman became pregnant.

Hormone changes can cause chemical changes in the brain that contribute to the onset of depression. Just as small changes in hormones can affect a woman's mood before her menstrual period, so these more severe changes in a new mother can lead to depression. Many women with PPD find that their depression gets much worse just before, or during, a period (see Premenstrual Syndrome).

Levels of thyroid hormones also plummet after childbirth (see Thyroid). The thyroid is a gland in the neck that helps regulate metabolism—that is, how the body uses and stores energy from foods eaten (see Metabolism). Low thyroid levels can cause symptoms that feel like depression—for example, mood swings, anxiety, and extreme fatigue. A woman's blood can be tested to see if a thyroid problem is causing her PPD and she can then be prescribed an appropriate thyroid medication.

Who is at risk?

Mothers of all ages and backgrounds can suffer from PPD. New mothers and mothers with more than one child are equally likely to get PPD. However, research suggests that women with a history of depression or a previous psychological disorder may be more at risk from PPD. Other factors can contribute to PPD, such as marital or relationship problems; a lack of support from one's partner, family, or friends; delivery complications for mother or baby; difficulties with the baby, such as health problems or feeding and sleeping difficulties; and severe premenstrual syndrome (PMS). A new mother is likely to feel tired and overwhelmed by the stresses of motherhood, which can also add to feelings of depression.

Treatment

If a new mother is depressed and having difficulty carrying out day-to-day activities, including looking after her baby, she should see her doctor immediately. If she is too anxious to leave the home, a home visit should be arranged. Postpartum depression, like other kinds of depression, can be treated and will go away eventually. The type of treatment depends on the severity of the depression.

Drug treatment

After diagnosing a severe case of PPD, a doctor may prescribe drug treatment—in the form of either tranquilizers or antidepressants (see Tranquilizers). Some drugs have unpleasant side effects, such as a dry mouth and drowsiness, which usually wear off as the drug is continually taken. However, drugs can make some people feel worse and it is important for a woman to return to her doctor to discuss alternatives if she is not feeling any better. A doctor should monitor the patient for any side effects and for her response to the medication (see Side Effects). It usually takes several weeks before most people start to notice a benefit from antidepressant drugs. These drugs are not habit-forming.

Therapy

A doctor may also suggest counseling or psychotherapy, either in conjunction with drug treatment or on its own if the depression is mild (see Psychotherapy). It can be very helpful for a woman with postpartum depression to talk about her illness and the way she feels. Counseling can be provided by a doctor, a health visitor, or a professional counselor (see Counseling)

A woman suffering from PPD needs as much help and support as possible from her family, her friends, and health professionals. Support can also be found from local mother-and-baby groups and self-help groups. A woman can help herself by trying to rest as much as possible, asking for help with household chores and child care, and talking to her partner, family, and friends about how she is feeling. Although a mother with PPD may find taking care of her baby difficult, it is usually not a good idea to separate mother and baby, as this can cause the depression to deepen.

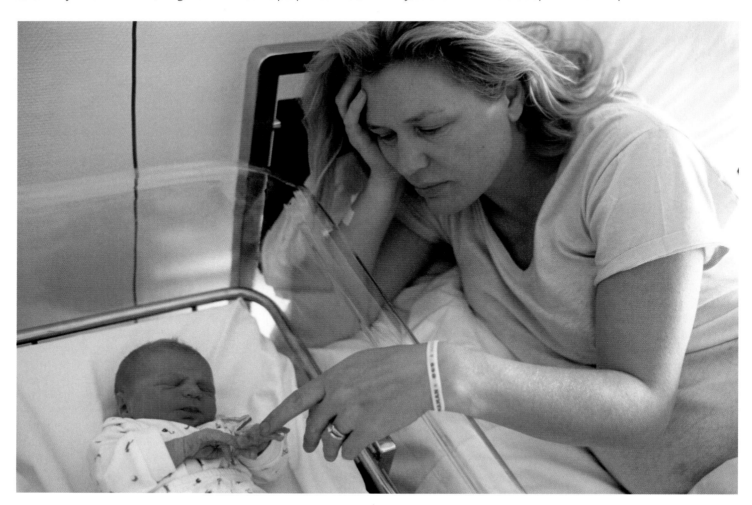

▲ *Some mothers may experience difficulties in bonding with their newborn babies, sometimes owing to the great fatigue felt after childbirth. If this difficulty persists, it can lead to overwhelming guilt and the onset of postpartum depression.*

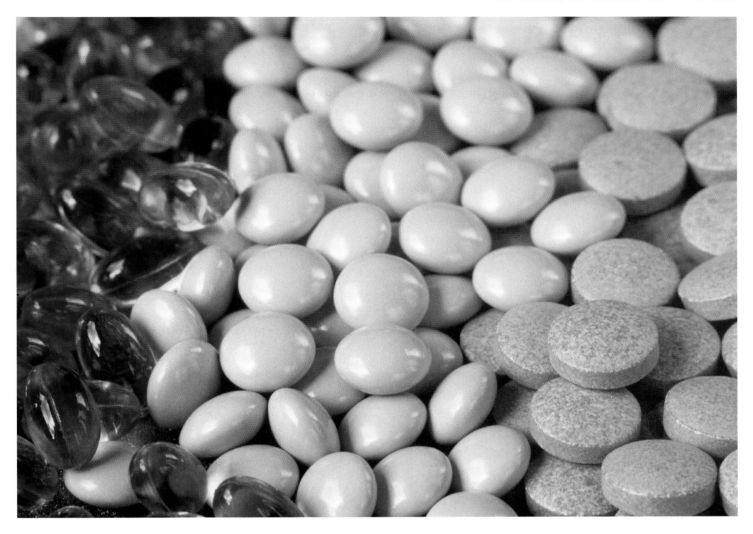

▲ *Vitamin supplements are thought to be beneficial for women suffering from postpartum depression. Some doctors particularly recommend taking 1,500 mg of calcium per day.*

It may also be helpful if a woman with PPD talks with other mothers to learn about their experiences. Maintaining a good diet, sometimes with a general vitamin supplement, and exercise can also be beneficial (see Diet; Exercise). Depression is often accompanied by aches and pains that are usually not a sign of a more serious illness. As the depression lifts, these pains will go away.

With proper medical help and support, a woman with mild symptoms of PPD will normally feel better in three to six months.

It is crucial for a woman with PPD to be patient and as kind to herself as possible. She needs to believe that she will, in time, get better. She also needs to have the reassurance that it is natural to feel overwhelmed by having a baby and that it can take some time to adjust to parenthood.

Recurrence

Postpartum depression can recur in future pregnancies, although there are few accurate studies of recurrence rates. Women with a history of PPD need extra support both during and after subsequent pregnancies and are advised to plan accordingly. They should be monitored by a health professional for any signs of depression.

Sometimes hormone patches are given after birth to counter the sudden drop in hormone levels.

Postpartum psychosis

Postpartum depression needs to be differentiated from postpartum psychosis, which is a very serious mental illness. This condition is rare, but it is extremely disabling and often requires hospitalization. Some hospitals have mother-and-baby units so that the bond between the mother and child can continue to be nurtured. The illness usually occurs in the first few weeks after childbirth. Women with postpartum psychosis can lose touch with reality and suffer from delusions and hallucinations. They may hear and see things that are not actually happening (see Hallucinations). Other symptoms include insomnia, confusion, agitation, and fluctuating moods (see Insomnia). Sometimes a woman suffering from postpartum psychosis can be at risk of harming herself or her baby. The precise cause of postpartum psychosis is not known. However, a previous history of depression alternating with episodes of mania can greatly increase the risk (see Bipolar Disorder). Women who have this illness need immediate medical attention. Treatment for PPD is usually in the form of drugs—antipsychotic and antidepressant medicines, or a mixture of both.

See also: **Depression; Hormones; Psychoses; Stress**

Post-traumatic stress disorder

Survivors of traumatic experiences may suffer recurring nightmares, overwhelming feelings of anger and fear, and a range of psychosomatic symptoms. Untreated, post-traumatic stress disorder (PTSD) may persist for months or even years, with damaging effects on the survivor's life.

Stressful situations trigger a particular reaction in humans and other living creatures. The hormone epinephrine (adrenaline) is released by the adrenal gland (see Hormones); the heart rate increases; the person becomes alert and experiences a temporary change in perception, so that he or she can ignore exhaustion or pain for a short time, and feels the emotions of fear or anger. This reaction, sometimes called the fight or flight response, is an essential survival mechanism. It prompts people to run from danger or turn around and fight, often calling on strength or speed that they had not realized they possessed.

Sometimes, however, this natural response is insufficient or inappropriate as a way of dealing with the danger at hand. Fighting or fleeing may even increase the danger. Feelings of fear may be overwhelming, causing the subject to freeze rather than act. At other times, the situation may be inescapable, as in the experience of victims of torture or child abuse. The normal fight or flight

Last year I was raped by an acquaintance. In some ways I was lucky; he didn't hurt me, although at the time I thought I was going to die. He has recently been sent to jail. However, I've begun to relive the rape over and over in my mind and I'm scared all the time. Why haven't I gotten over it by now?

It's not uncommon to experience such symptoms, particularly if something has occurred to remind you of the event—for example, the end of a criminal trial. Talking through your experience will help; if you can't share your fears with friends or relatives, contact a rape survivors' group. Psychotherapy or counseling may also help.

My son takes pride in being in the army. He saw combat in the Gulf War but hasn't suffered any bad effects. Is he right when he says PTSD is another name for shirking?

Not everyone in a combat situation gets PTSD afterward, although the likelihood increases with factors such as the seriousness of the conflict. The condition is a well-documented effect of battle, sometimes suffered by the bravest fighters. It is far from being an excuse to avoid combat; its disabling effects can frustrate those who want to return to the front line.

My father is a firefighter. A few months ago he saw two of his co-workers die in an industrial fire. Since then he has started drinking and has bursts of anger, but won't talk about it. Is this just a phase?

Your father's behavior sounds typical of the early stages of PTSD. Guilt over the inability to save lives is a strong factor in PTSD. He may continue to have these and other symptoms for a long time. His employers should urge counseling to help him to come to terms with his dreadful experience.

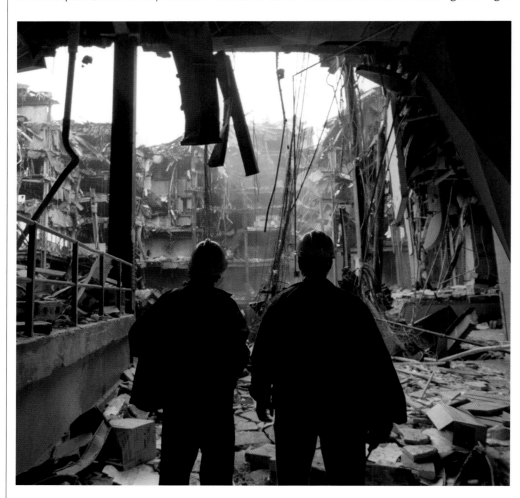

▲ *The attack on the twin towers in New York on September 11, 2001, killed and maimed innocent people; it also led to post-traumatic stress disorder in the injured, and in members of the rescue services following this catastrophic act of terrorism.*

response is not allowed an outlet and the victim loses any sense of control over the situation.

The result can be that the survivors of severe trauma may recover well from any physical injuries only to suffer psychological effects for a long time afterward. Collectively called post-traumatic stress disorder (PTSD), these psychological effects can take the form of nightmares and hallucinations; depression and a general feeling of emotional numbness; outbursts of violent anger; physical symptoms, such as an inability to talk or move that has no obvious physical cause; and overwhelming feelings of helplessness and loss of control (see Depression; Dreaming; Hallucinations). PTSD sufferers often believe their personality has been completely changed by the trauma they have experienced; in some cases they may even feel as if it has been annihilated.

A new name for an old illness

"Post-traumatic stress disorder" is a fairly recent term, first used in the American Psychiatric Association's manual in 1980. However, the condition it describes has been recognized for many years. In the late 19th century, the French neurologist Jean-Martin Charcot, studying a strange disease known at the time as hysteria, cataloged symptoms in his patients that would be familiar to modern specialists in PTSD. Charcot's research inspired, among others, Sigmund Freud, whose book *The Etiology of Hysteria* put forward the idea that hysteria in his female patients arose from their experience of childhood sexual abuse, a theory he later rejected, but it has been revived by some modern psychotherapists.

In Britain, in the aftermath of World War I, a similar set of symptoms was found in men who had fought in the trenches. At first it was attributed to concussion from exploding shells—hence the term "shell shock." However, it soon became obvious that the condition affected many soldiers who had not been physically injured and that it was primarily psychological. One estimate was that mental breakdown accounted for 40 percent of British casualties.

Some doctors attributed shell shock, which was also called "combat neurosis" and then "combat fatigue," to weakness and cowardice. However, the British psychologist W. H. R. Rivers argued that it was a genuine illness. He went on to have some success using psychoanalysis in the treatment of sufferers. One of his best-known patients was the war poet Siegfried Sassoon, who returned to the battlefield after being treated, but went on reliving the horror of his war experiences for the rest of his life.

The study of PTSD in the United States was pioneered by Abram Kardiner, a psychiatrist working for the Veterans' Administration in the 1920s. Kardiner's work with sufferers of combat neurosis in the wake of World War I and during World War II led to the conclusion that anyone could suffer psychological breakdown under great stress, and that this disorder and its symptoms were entirely predictable in situations such as combat. However, little was done to investigate the long-term aftereffects of trauma until the Vietnam war in the 1960s and 1970s, when veterans' groups prompted studies into such lasting psychological trauma as a legacy of war.

More recent studies of trauma survivors have suggested the need for a division of post-traumatic stress disorder into at least two separate forms: type I, or simple PTSD, a reaction to a single traumatic event such as an assault or a natural disaster; and type II, or complex PTSD, a more crippling disorder arising from prolonged, repeated, inescapable trauma. Complex PTSD is characteristic of those who have experienced torture or imprisonment in brutal conditions. It is a description that may apply to a wide range of sufferers, from victims of childhood abuse to survivors of the Holocaust.

Symptoms

Typical of PTSD is a general feeling of anxiety, combined with fears relating to the trauma experienced. Sufferers have a higher than normal base level of arousal; in other words, they are constantly alert to any potential dangers, are easily startled, and will react strongly to stimuli that recall the trauma; for example, a car backfiring may sound like an explosion on the battlefield.

These symptoms of hyperarousal tend to be found along with sleep disorders. Sufferers take a long time to fall asleep; they wake often in the night; and their sleep is more easily disturbed by noise (see Sleep and Sleep Problems).

Intrusive, unwanted reminders of the trauma itself are the most obvious symptoms of PTSD and appear the first few days and weeks after the trauma has ended. Survivors may be obsessed with the trauma, repeatedly dreaming about it during sleep and experiencing flashbacks during waking hours. These nightmares and flashbacks are unlike memories of normal events, which are modified as time passes. The sufferer finds it impossible to describe memories of the trauma and put them into perspective as part of her or his life story, but experiences them in the form of vivid images and sensations, as if reliving the trauma all over again.

These intrusive memories have an emotional intensity that other memories lack, being accompanied by the same overwhelming feelings experienced at that time of the trauma. Repetitiveness is another characteristic: trauma memories persist without changing or developing, while survivors may compulsively repeat patterns of behavior relating to the trauma itself, for example by irrational risk-taking in battle. Traumatized children may play obsessive, monotonously repetitive games that act out the experience they have suffered. The repetition compulsion may be an attempt to reexperience the event in order to regain control over it (see Complexes and Compulsions).

Intrusive symptoms tend to become less frequent with time. Studies of rape victims have found that the symptoms start to diminish after about three to six months, although many sufferers still had nonspecific feelings of fear and anxiety for as long as a year afterward. Trauma-related symptoms may also resurface for many years when prompted by a reminder such as an anniversary.

When intrusive symptoms diminish, however, they are replaced by constrictive ones. Constriction can be an essential survival tactic in times of inescapable danger. When action against the danger is impossible, one natural reaction is altered consciousness: an abrupt switch from feelings of terror or fury to a detached calm, a trancelike or hypnotic state called dissociation. The sufferer continues to be aware of what is happening but no longer has an appropriate emotional reaction to events and often becomes completely passive. The person may even feel that he or she is dreaming or observing the trauma from a distance rather than actually experiencing it.

Dissociation protects people from feelings of pain that would otherwise be unendurable. It is not unlike an involuntary form of self-hypnosis, although prisoners have been known to teach each other the secret of entering a trancelike state during episodes of torture or extreme hunger (see Hypnosis).

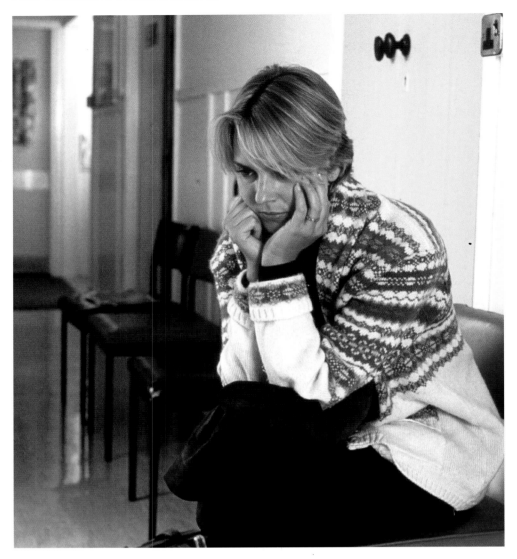

The terrible, senseless death of a child may lead to overwhelming guilt in the parents. Their feelings of helplessness and loss translate into anger, nightmares, and numbness—all signs of PTSD due to severe trauma.

People differ in their ability to dissociate naturally; some may resort to alcohol or drug abuse to produce the same emotional numbing (see Alcoholism; Drug Abuse). Notoriously, this played a part in enabling U.S. soldiers to face falling morale during the Vietnam war. Children usually find it easier to dissociate than adults, and it is extremely common for abused children to survive their ordeals by altering their consciousness in this way.

Although constrictive behavior can be useful at the time of trauma, it prevents the experience from becoming part of everyday consciousness. This mental numbness may persist as a feeling of emptiness and of going through the motions of living rather than properly experiencing life. PTSD sufferers may lead severely restricted lives because they avoid any experiences that may evoke the original trauma, and they lose the ability to plan for the future and take the initiative. Rational thinking may be replaced by reliance on lucky charms and superstitions to influence events. Those who use narcotics to numb their feelings are likely to develop an addiction rather than deal with reality (see Narcotics).

This constriction is self-perpetuating: by avoiding risks and opportunities to take action, sufferers pass up the chance to regain some control over their lives. In the long term, the resulting depression may lead to breakdown or they may even try to commit suicide (see Nervous Breakdown; Suicide).

People at risk

Anyone experiencing serious trauma is at risk of suffering post-traumatic stress disorder later on. Survivors of natural disasters such as earthquakes or fires, or those who live through brutalities such as war, torture, imprisonment, or domestic or street violence, rarely come through completely unscathed. However, this fact does not imply that PTSD is inevitable or that it always follows the same pattern. The strongest factor affecting the occurrence of PTSD is the severity of the trauma. A national study of veterans of Vietnam found that more than a third of those who had been involved in heavy combat still suffered the symptoms of PTSD 15 years later; only 9 percent of veterans who had fought in light to moderate combat conditions were affected.

However, the form that symptoms take is influenced by personality: people who were aggressive before the trauma may have symptoms of anger and violence; those who have high moral standards are more prone to depressive symptoms.

Some people have less resilience than others when faced with traumatic experiences; everyone has a different breaking point. A few individuals are exceptionally resilient. Typically, they are alert and active, sociable, and skillful communicators, with a highly developed sense of being in command of their own destiny. Psychologists call this resilience a strong locus of control. In a dangerous situation resilient people are more likely to take constructive action by cooperating with others and are less likely to be paralyzed by fear. They also seem less likely to suffer from PTSD than others facing the same or an equivalent trauma. Social ties of some sort, a sense of comradeship in a combat unit, or close friendships in prison camps help people not only to survive the trauma but also to mitigate the worst effects of PTSD.

Those most likely to develop the symptoms of PTSD are people who react to trauma by freezing or dissociating, or alternatively by taking reckless, individualistic action rather than cooperating. Symptoms tend to be worse in survivors who feel guilt for failing to help or save comrades or relatives; experiencing the death of friends or family members is one of the events most likely to lead to severe, enduring PTSD (see Grief). The highest risk of PTSD arises when a survivor has taken part in violence. Veterans of Vietnam who had

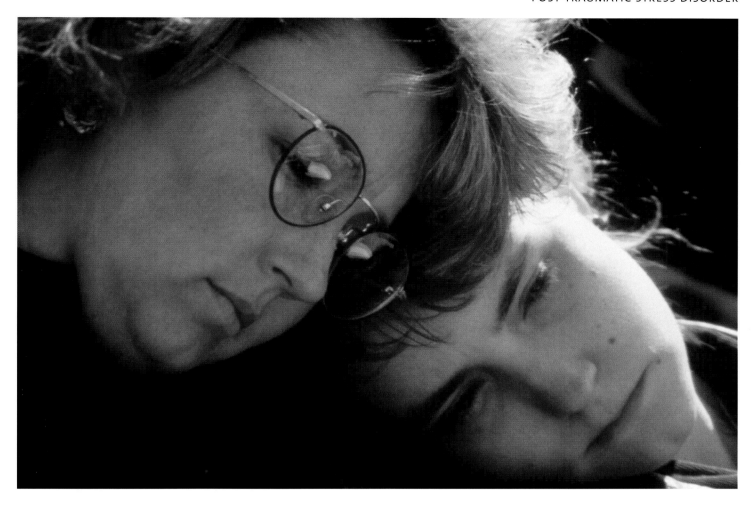

▲ *People with PTSD must share the memories of their trauma if they are to overcome it. Emotional support from family and friends can be a lifeline back to normality.*

individually committed atrocities as well as experiencing the stress of combat suffered the worst symptoms.

The length of the trauma, and whether it is a single event or a continuing series of attacks and restrictions, is also an important factor in the severity and duration of PTSD. Survivors of prisoner-of-war camps and of concentration camps in World War II were found to be still experiencing nightmares and flashbacks 40 years after the end of their ordeal.

Treatment and outlook
The fundamental experience of PTSD is isolation and loss of control. Treatment of the condition is based on restoring control to the sufferer: in Kardiner's words, helping the patient "complete the job that he is trying to do spontaneously," and reviving social relationships and trust in others. This may involve working with a therapist or within a self-help group or survivors' organization, where people who have been through similar traumas share experiences and offer support (see Group Therapy).

Specific symptoms such as panic attacks may respond to behavioral therapy such as relaxation training or desensitization (see Behavior Therapy). Antidepressants and minor tranquilizers can also prove useful in treating sleep disorders, anxiety, and intrusive symptoms in the short term (see Hypnotic Drugs). The sense of achievement provided by overcoming these symptoms can help the sufferer to regain a feeling of power over his or her own life.

It is important that the person suffering from PTSD can find a safe environment, preferably with support from family and close friends who show that they take his or her experiences seriously and are prepared to listen. A form of psychotherapy such as cognitive therapy may be helpful to enable victims to acknowledge the trauma they have been through, incorporate it into their other memories, and mourn for their own suffering. Some survivors of trauma regain self-esteem by taking part in relevant social action, for example, by working for a rape crisis center, campaigning on behalf of war veterans, or providing testimony on torture to human rights groups.

Survivors of a single traumatic event can take a few simple steps to limit the symptoms of PTSD, by avoiding the use of drugs or alcohol to blot out memories of the experience, by reconstructing the event in words and discussing it as much as possible, and by ensuring that they have a sympathetic social network of support. Survivors of more serious and prolonged traumas may take many years to recover, however, and may find their symptoms recurring even after a long period of remission under stress or on anniversaries of the event.

See also: Anxiety; Child abuse; Counseling; Hysteria; Psychosomatic problems; Psychotherapy; Rape; Stress

Posture

Is the traditional military-style posture the best one to aim for?

In general, yes. The ideal is a straight spine with the back of the shoulders and the back of the buttocks in line, the shoulders drawn well back, and the chest pushed slightly forward. The chin should be tucked in and the eyes looking straight ahead.

What is the best posture to adopt during pregnancy?

The increasingly large and heavy forward bulge in the abdomen during pregnancy can become a source of back strain and great discomfort unless it is managed properly. Many women tend to bend backward so that the weight is carried by the spine rather than the abdominal muscles because they think that this is more likely to preserve their figure. Instead, it is likely to give them backache. The best course is to let both the spine and the abdominal muscles bear the load, by holding your posture as close to the normal straight-backed position as possible. If you have prepared your abdominal muscles by appropriate exercises, they will be strong enough to support the extra weight without sagging.

If you have bad posture habits when you are young, will this cause back trouble when you are older?

Yes. All the joints of your body suffer wear and tear over the years, but the joints in the lower part of the body—feet, ankles, knees, hips, and lumbar spine—are under even greater strain because they have to support the whole weight of your body. In later life, these joints are the most likely to become painfully arthritic. You can help prevent this by keeping your weight down and maintaining good posture so that the joints do not have to suffer unnecessary strain.

"Posture" is the term used to refer to the way people stand and move about. The sedentary nature of so many modern occupations has contributed to bad posture and many internal and back problems.

The normal upright stance that humans have adopted has taken millions of years to evolve, and the process is briefly repeated in the life of each new baby, who at first can move about only by crawling on hands and knees. The restricted positions adopted in the uterus are changed gradually by the baby's natural stretching and kicking reflexes, until at the age of 12 to 15 months he or she is strong and well-balanced enough to stand upright.

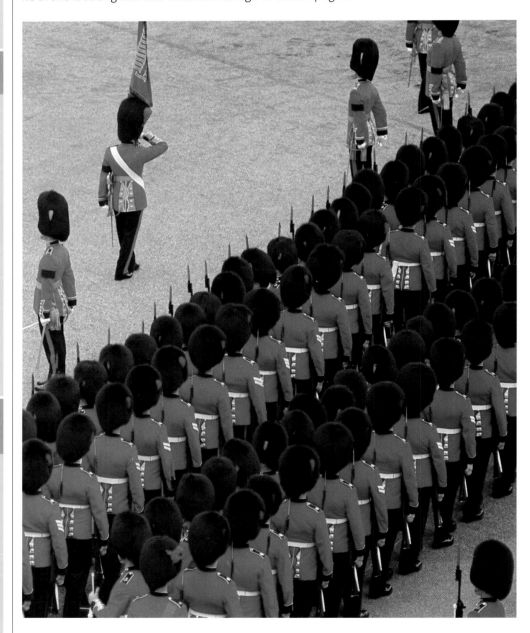

▲ *The military stance is everyone's idea of good posture—and indeed it makes a great deal of sense: a straight spine with the shoulders back, chest forward, and head erect.*

Posture and the force of gravity

The overwhelming physical force to which the human body is subject is the earth's natural pull, or gravity. The body's center of gravity—the point where its weight is balanced—is in the lower back and pelvis. Good posture is primarily a matter of efficiently balancing the body weight around this point (see Balance). This must be done not only when a person is still but when he or she walks, sits, runs, works, plays games, and so on. Whatever movements are made, the weight on all sides of that point has to be equal, otherwise a person will tend to topple over (see Movement).

Because this area of the back is the focus of so many of the body's movements, and because it bears the brunt of any lifting, it is particularly vulnerable to injury, damage, and disorders.

Muscle control

The body's erect posture is achieved and maintained only by a fine muscular adjustment that is concentrated around its center of gravity and supported by the ligaments of the spine (see Spinal Cord).

Muscles can act only by shortening or contracting, not by stretching (see Muscles). Therefore, to reverse a movement, another muscle has to act in the opposite direction. Each muscle can also work together with other muscles to produce a balanced movement by pulling at the same time, but not with full power.

Well-balanced movements require not only muscular power but relaxation in those muscles that act in the opposite direction. Economy and precision of muscular effort, which are essential to good posture, improve when stress is removed. A person who is mentally relaxed will as a result be physically relaxed and therefore able to stand and move well (see Mind-Body Therapy).

The role of the nervous system

Posture is not simply a matter of muscle control. The muscles themselves have to be controlled, and this is done by the nervous system. In a child who is learning to stand and walk for the first time, this process of keeping balance is a conscious one. However, soon habit patterns develop and the action becomes automatic (see Nervous System).

Messages indicating the position of various parts of the body in space, and in relation to each other, are transmitted from nerve endings in the skin and in the muscles along to the spinal cord and the brain. Signals are then sent to activate the appropriate muscles in the body for any necessary movement or change in position.

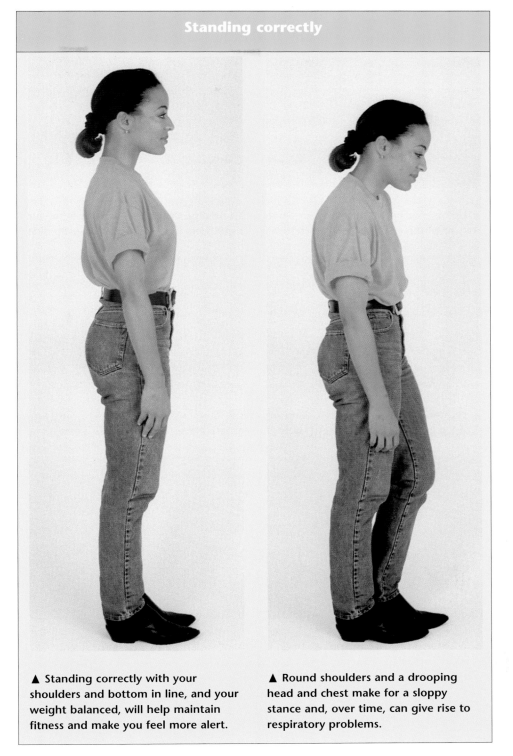

Standing correctly

▲ Standing correctly with your shoulders and bottom in line, and your weight balanced, will help maintain fitness and make you feel more alert.

▲ Round shoulders and a drooping head and chest make for a sloppy stance and, over time, can give rise to respiratory problems.

Thus poor balance, abnormal posture, muscular weakness, and poor coordination of movements may each be due to disorders of the nervous system or disorders of the muscles (see Coordination). The connection is such that if, for example, a muscle loses its nerve supply, it can no longer contract sufficiently and so begins to waste away.

Good and bad posture

Apart from disorders of balance, people's posture may be either good or bad. Good posture depends largely on keeping all the postural

Simple exercises to improve your posture

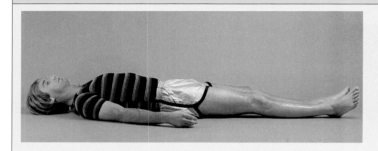

▲ Lie on your back and relax your whole body. Breathe deeply. Start from this position and return to it if you get tired.

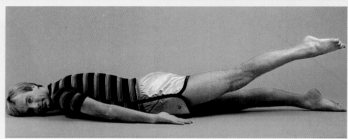

▲ Turn onto your front and practice straight leg raising from this position, first lifting each leg alternately, as before.

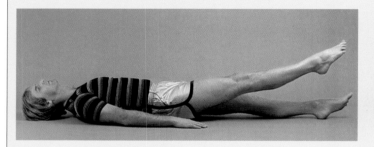

▲ Tighten and relax your buttock muscles. Rest, then raise each leg in turn with the knee straight. Repeat four times.

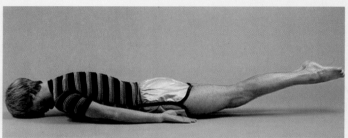

▲ Now raise both legs. If you feel any muscle strain doing these exercises, adopt the rest position immediately.

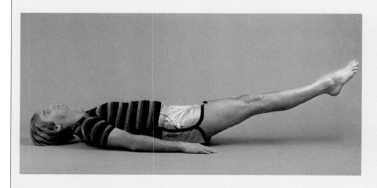

▲ When you feel strong enough to do it without strain, try to raise both legs together, still keeping them straight.

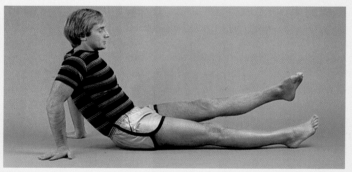

▲ To strengthen the foot and ankle, move each foot in turn in a circular motion, first clockwise, then counterclockwise.

muscles of the body toned and balanced. Good posture requires the conscious effort of maintaining balance at all times, and of getting adequate exercise in order to keep all the joints and muscles healthy (see Exercise). To ensure correct posture and avoid strains and unnecessary accidents, posture training is needed. The appropriate exercises can be enjoyable and help people learn how the body works and how to take care of it. Maintaining good posture or correcting bad posture not only will transform the appearance but will substantially benefit health and make the person feel fresher at the end of the day.

Bad posture has specific ill effects. Bad stance and movement can affect the hip joints and the lowest joint of the back, which are more prone to developing arthritis in later life (see Arthritis). Lower-back pain, slipped disk, and sciatica are also more likely to occur (see

Lower-Back Pain; Sciatica; Slipped Disk). Obesity increases the likelihood of bad posture because the extra weight increases the strain on the body's muscles (see Obesity).

Another disorder caused by poor posture is foot strain. This often occurs in people whose jobs involve long periods of standing and walking. The strain happens because they are standing and walking incorrectly and too much strain is placed on the ligaments and bones of the foot arches, causing pain. This may be avoided by doing simple exercises to strengthen the feet and ankles (see Feet).

See also: Alexander technique; Back and backache; Bones; Ligaments; Pelvis; Pregnancy; Relaxation; Weight; Yoga

Preeclampsia

Questions and Answers

I am 36 weeks' pregnant and my fingers and ankles are swollen and puffy, especially in the mornings. Could I have preeclampsia?

Swelling and puffiness are common during pregnancy because the body is less efficient at getting rid of fluid from the tissues. On its own, swelling is not a symptom of preeclampsia, which is suspected only if two of three of the symptoms (fluid retention, raised blood pressure, and protein in the urine) exist. If your next prenatal checkup is not due for several days, however, and you are worried, ask to see your obstetrician to set your mind at rest. Both preeclampsia and eclampsia can develop rapidly, so it is best to be cautious.

Is it true that taking half an aspirin each day may reduce the chances of developing preeclampsia?

Some studies indicate this, but the results are not conclusive. Aspirin can have its own dangers for some people and should be taken regularly only on a doctor's advice and under medical supervision. Other studies suggest that a high-protein diet reduces the risk of developing preeclampsia, but, again, radical changes in diet should be made only on the advice of the doctor. The best advice is to eat sensibly and get sufficient rest, since rest is believed to improve blood flow to the fetus.

If I get preeclampsia, will I be likely to have a cesarean section?

Not if the condition has been treated successfully. However, if it persists and there is a risk of eclampsia, a cesarean section will be done rather than risk the health of mother and baby. A cesarean section may also be advised if the mother's preeclampsia has been cured but she still has high blood pressure, because the process of labor itself raises blood pressure.

This serious condition can develop very suddenly during late pregnancy. It occurs in 5 to 7 percent of pregnancies and is more common in some areas of the world, including the southeastern parts of the United States, than others.

Preeclampsia (preeclamptic toxemia, PET; or proteinuric hypertension) is a condition that occurs only during the later stages of pregnancy, generally from 24 weeks onward. It can be mild or severe, but if it is left untreated it can quickly develop into a very dangerous and sometimes fatal condition, eclampsia.

Symptoms of preeclampsia

The main symptoms of preeclampsia include a significant rise in blood pressure (even if the reading is still within the normal range); puffiness of the face, hands, and feet (especially in the mornings) caused by the retention of fluid (see Edema); and protein in the urine (proteinuria). Taken separately, all of these symptoms are common during pregnancy, and one symptom on its own is not generally serious. However, when two or more of these symptoms are present at one time, doctors will suspect preeclampsia. Other possible symptoms include unusual weight gain, morning sickness

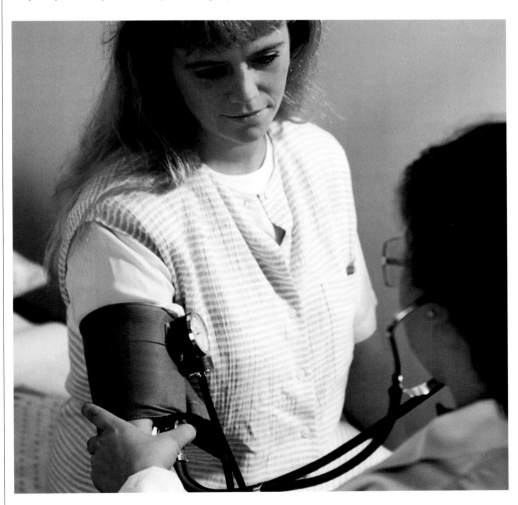

▲ *A full-term pregnant woman has her blood pressure taken by a nurse. Such tests are vital, particularly during the latter stages of pregnancy, when a high reading may indicate the presence of preeclampsia.*

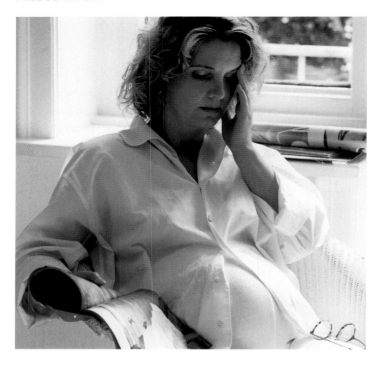

▲ *Headaches are common during pregnancy, as are morning sickness and fatigue. A combination of such symptoms, particularly if they persist, may indicate preeclampsia.*

that continues into late pregnancy (see Morning Sickness), abdominal pain, constant headache, blurred vision, and visual disturbances.

Causes

Much medical research into the causes of preeclampsia has been done, but, as yet, no definitive cause has been found. The condition may be partly genetic; women whose close relatives have suffered from it are more likely to develop it, although not all women with a family history of preeclampsia do so. Another theory suggests that the condition stems from an abnormality in the way a woman's body responds to pregnancy. Women with autoimmune diseases seem to have an increased incidence of the condition.

Preeclampsia is also more common in first pregnancies; multiple pregnancies; women whose diet is poor before and during pregnancy; women who have had diabetes, high blood pressure (see Blood Pressure), or chronic kidney disease (see Kidneys and Kidney Diseases) before pregnancy; women who live in poverty; women under 20 or over 40 years of age; and women who abuse alcohol or drugs, or who smoke heavily during pregnancy (see Smoking). However, preeclampsia also affects some women who do not fit into any of the above categories.

Diagnosis and treatment

Preeclampsia is most commonly identified during a woman's regular prenatal checkups (see Prenatal Care). These checkups include regular blood pressure and urine checks, as well as a regular weight check. If a woman has more than one of the possible symptoms of preeclampsia, the doctor will carry out further checks.

In mild cases, rest in bed, usually in the hospital, may be all the treatment that is needed. Drugs may also be given to reduce blood pressure, and the doctor will keep a very close eye on the patient. If

the condition is diagnosed early and kept under control until the baby is born, preeclampsia usually disappears with no complications during the first week after delivery. If it does not respond to treatment, stronger drugs may be given. Since the condition originates from a disorder in the placenta, however, the one certain cure is to deliver the baby, and thus also the placenta. If the woman is near term, the doctor may decide to deliver the baby early, either by inducing the birth or by cesarean section.

Dangers of preeclampsia

Preeclampsia can lead to premature separation of the placenta, restricting the fetus's growth and leading to low birth weight. The main danger, however, is that untreated preeclampsia can quickly lead to eclampsia. The term "eclampsia" means "sudden development," and the condition can develop in a matter of hours. However, eclampsia is extremely rare; it occurs in only 0.2 percent of pregnancies.

Symptoms of eclampsia

A woman with eclampsia will have some or all of the symptoms of preeclampsia, together with the symptoms of eclampsia itself, which include a very high temperature of up to 104°F (40°C), coma, convulsions, mental dullness, blurred vision, confusion, muscle twitching, and breathing difficulties.

About 3 percent of mothers and 15 percent of fetuses with eclampsia die every year. However, even if eclampsia is not fatal, the possible effects of the condition in the mother include major epileptic seizures, cerebral hemorrhage, pulmonary edema (accumulation of fluid in the lungs), kidney failure, possible blindness if the retina is damaged, necrosis (tissue death) of the liver, hypofibrinogenemia (deficiency of the blood clotting factor fibrinogen), and hemolysis (breakdown of red blood cells). The baby may suffer from retarded growth and brain damage.

Diagnosis and treatment

Eclampsia is treated with anticonvulsant (usually magnesium sulfate) and antihypertensive drugs. If convulsions occur, the medical staff will keep a close watch to ensure that the woman does not stop breathing. An endotracheal tube is sometimes inserted down the throat to assist in breathing. Because delivery of the baby brings an instant end to the condition, the birth may be induced or a cesarean section undertaken as soon as the mother's condition is stable. Recent research suggests that the antioxidant vitamins C and E may be valuable in reducing the risk of eclampsia (see Antioxidants).

Prevention

It is not possible to prevent preeclampsia, but the risks can be minimized. Since the condition can develop very quickly, all pregnant women should have regular prenatal checkups. If a woman develops symptoms of preeclampsia, she should contact her obstetrician immediately. She should avoid smoking, alcohol, and illegal drugs, take only medication prescribed by the doctor, and check with him or her before taking any over-the-counter remedies. A woman who has diabetes, kidney disease, or high blood pressure should ask to see an obstetrician who specializes in high-risk pregnancies from the start of the pregnancy (see Obstetrics).

See also: **Cesarean birth; Fetus; Placenta; Pregnancy; Swellings; Urinary tract and disorders**

Pregnancy

Questions and Answers

I think I might be pregnant. How soon would it be worthwhile to do a pregnancy test?

Pregnancy tests are now more sensitive. Most of the older tests were not reliable until five or six weeks after the last period, but now a test may be possible within a week after conception.

What can I do to prevent indigestion during pregnancy?

The hormones of pregnancy, and later pressure of the uterus on the stomach, tend to make the digestive acid pass back from the stomach into the esophagus, where it causes a burning sensation. This acid can be mopped up by drinking milk, eating small frequent meals, and taking antacids. Another way to prevent heartburn at night is to raise the head of the bed.

Can you prevent stretch marks from forming during pregnancy?

Some women, especially very fair women, seem more likely to get stretch marks, which form on the breasts, stomach, and thighs. Once the baby is born, the marks will lose their reddish color and eventually fade, but will never entirely disappear. Very little can be done to prevent them, although some women believe that a little olive oil rubbed into the skin every day helps.

My husband is worried about making love to me now that I am pregnant. Is he right to be?

No. You should continue to make love for as long as you feel comfortable enough to enjoy it. Occasionally, women who have had many miscarriages are advised to avoid making love in the first three months of pregnancy, but there is no absolute proof that this makes them any less likely to miscarry.

In pregnancy, changes occur in the mother's body that are designed to meet the needs of the growing fetus. For most women it is an exciting and happy time; modern prenatal care has also made it much safer.

Pregnancy is the remarkable and highly complex process between conception and labor and lasts on average 38 weeks. Because the date of conception is often not known exactly, it is easier to date the pregnancy from the first day of the last menstrual period, which is usually about two weeks before conception (see Menstruation), making a total of 40 weeks.

The first signs

The first sign of pregnancy is usually a missed period, although this can be caused by other conditions. However, if intercourse without contraception has taken place, pregnancy is the most likely cause (see Contraception; Intercourse).

Other early symptoms include a sense of fullness and tingling in the breasts and an urgent need to pass urine more frequently. Many women suffer from nausea, and even vomiting in early pregnancy. Although this is popularly called morning sickness, it can come at any time of day. It is often aggravated by preparing food. A cup of herbal tea and a dry cracker first thing in the morning can sometimes help, and it is sensible to eat small amounts of nongreasy food at fairly frequent intervals through the day rather than large infrequent meals.

If a woman thinks she is pregnant

A woman should do a home pregnancy test as soon as she suspects that she might be pregnant. The pregnancy test will detect the presence or absence of a hormone called human chorionic gonadotropin, which is produced by the developing egg and excreted in the mother's urine. Simple home pregnancy tests are available from drugstores. If the woman carries out the test herself she should still consult her family doctor if the result is positive. If she does not wish to have her baby, she may need to find an adoption center, or talk to her doctor. If the fetus is not developing normally, she may have a spontaneous abortion.

Once a woman's pregnancy is confirmed, her obstetrician will arrange for her care during pregnancy and plan for her to go to the hospital where the obstetrician has admitting rights. She will also need to make office visits, probably on a monthly basis throughout the first 28 weeks of

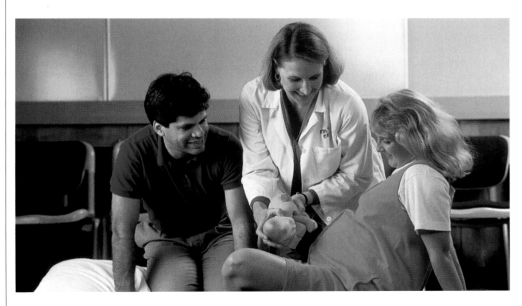

▲ *Fathers are welcome at prenatal classes, where they learn how to help their partners.*

Questions and Answers

I often feel faint when I lie on my back. Why?

This usually happens only late in pregnancy when the baby's weight in the uterus can press on a large blood vessel, the inferior vena cava, and decrease the blood supply to your heart and brain. If you feel faint, turn over onto your side and the faintness should soon pass.

Since I have become pregnant I need to urinate more frequently. Does this mean I have cystitis?

That is a possibility, and your urine will be tested at the doctor's office for any signs of infection. However, it's more likely that your uterus and bladder are competing for space in the pelvis and so your bladder feels full sooner. In the middle part of pregnancy, when the uterus has grown out of your pelvis, you will probably return to normal, but in the last weeks the baby's head often presses on the bladder, and you will find again that you need to urinate more frequently.

Is it true that a woman "blossoms" during pregnancy, and if so, why?

Pregnancy certainly suits some women very well. This is because the hormones of pregnancy often improve a woman's complexion and make her feel warmer, so that she has rosy cheeks. Even more important is the sense of well-being some women feel at this time, which is thought to be related to increased production of hormones called steroids.

My mother tells me that now that I'm pregnant I must eat for two, but I don't want to be fat after the birth. How much should I eat?

Your mother is wrong—you burn up your food more efficiently and use up less energy yourself as you become less active late in pregnancy. You simply need to eat a normal sensible diet with plenty of milk products, fish, meat, and fruit. Your obstetrician will keep an eye on your weight gain.

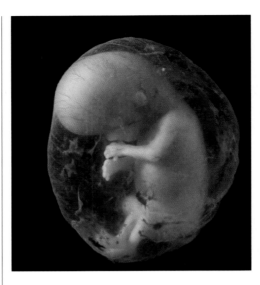

▲ *This 11-week-old fetus, although only 2 in. (5 cm) long, is recognizably human.*

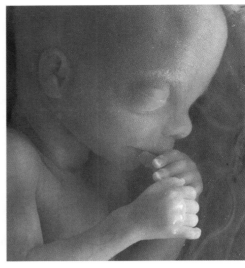

▲ *By four months the fetus has developed eyebrows, but the eyelids are still fused.*

pregnancy, then every two weeks until 36 weeks, and thereafter weekly until the baby is born. Obviously these arrangements have to be flexible to allow for any unusual circumstances.

Prenatal visits not only involve checks and tests to see if the mother and baby are both healthy, but may also include classes on baby care and preparation for labor and childbirth. Most courses will also include at least one session for prospective fathers to advise them on how to help their partners during pregnancy and labor and after the birth.

Minor discomforts

During pregnancy a woman may suffer from several minor discomforts which, although mostly trivial, can cause her some anxiety.

Nausea: Feelings of nausea noticed early in pregnancy usually continue until about 16 weeks. If they are severe enough to be incapacitating, the obstetrician may prescribe medicine that can help.

Vaginal discharge: Women have an increased vaginal discharge in pregnancy. Unless the discharge is offensive or irritating, it does not require medical attention (see Vaginal Discharge).

Backache and cramp: Muscular aches and pains may present a problem as the pregnancy advances. A pregnant woman instinctively tends to throw her shoulders back in an attempt to counteract the weight of the growing uterus, and this can put undue strain on the back. Improved posture and comfortable, low-heeled shoes may relieve it (see Posture). Leg cramps are most common in late pregnancy and may be quite troublesome at night (see Cramp). They can sometimes be relieved by gently stretching the affected muscle.

Constipation and heartburn: Both are commonly experienced during a pregnancy. They are side effects of the hormone progesterone, which relaxes the smooth muscle fibers in the uterus. However, its action is not confined to the growing uterus; it has effects throughout the mother's body. It affects the intestines, making them sluggish (see Constipation), as well as the sphincter muscle at the opening from the esophagus into the stomach. This can allow the contents of the stomach to be regurgitated and cause heartburn. A mild antacid can help (see Heartburn).

Hemorrhoids: These are fairly common in pregnancy because the blood flow to and from the woman's legs and pelvis is partially obstructed by pressure from the baby and the uterus. Straining through constipation can aggravate the problem (see Hemorrhoids).

Varicose veins: These may become worse during pregnancy, owing to the effect of progesterone on the blood vessels. They may also appear for the first time. Maternity support hose can help to prevent their formation, and this should be put on before the woman actually gets out of bed in the morning. Women with varicose veins should avoid standing still for long periods; it is better to walk around to keep the circulation going. When the woman is sitting, she should prop up her feet on a stool or a low chair (see Varicose Veins).

Edema: This condition is caused by excess amounts of water in the pregnant mother's body. This fluid accumulates in certain areas, creating swelling, particularly around the ankles and the feet (see Edema). Mild cases of edema are fairly common in later pregnancy; a low-salt diet and plenty of rest with the feet up should help. However, if edema is associated with an increase in blood pressure and protein in the urine, special treatment will be necessary, since these symptoms could indicate preeclamptic toxemia, which is a very serious condition (see Preeclampsia).

Skin changes: As the pregnancy proceeds, stretch marks can appear across the abdomen, thighs, and breasts. Little can be done to prevent these from developing , but they will usually fade after the baby has been born (see Stretch Marks).

Changes in the uterus and breasts

A pregnancy is divided into three trimesters of about 13 weeks each. In the first trimester, the uterus grows rapidly but remains within the pelvic cavity. It is during the second trimester, when the uterus moves up into the abdominal cavity, that a woman first becomes obviously pregnant (see Uterus).

By about 22 weeks the upper edge of the uterus, or fundus, reaches the navel, and at 36 weeks most of the abdominal cavity is occupied. The intestines are pushed upward and sideways so they press on the stomach and diaphragm. Because of pressure on the diaphragm, the lungs cannot expand fully, and many women find themselves short of breath quite regularly (see Diaphragm).

At about 22 weeks into a first pregnancy and 18 weeks in subsequent pregnancies the mother will start to feel her baby's movements. The fetal heartbeat is usually audible through a stethoscope by about 24 weeks (see Stethoscope).

The main change that a woman notices in the breasts during pregnancy is that they grow larger in preparation for feeding. The areola, the ring of darker skin around the nipple, becomes larger and darker in color and a secondary areola appears, which helps to improve the strength of the skin.

From about 12 weeks of a pregnancy the breasts produce a protein-rich substance called colostrum, and in the last few weeks this fluid may leak. Colostrum provides all the nutritional needs of the newborn baby until the milk appears on the third day after birth (see Breasts).

Prenatal care

At each office visit for a prenatal checkup, the pregnant mother will be weighed, her blood pressure measured, and a urine

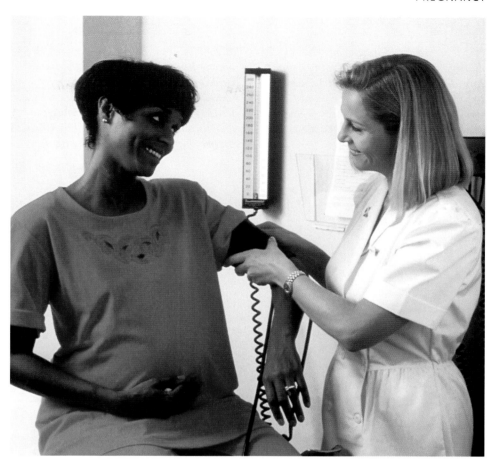

▲ *Expectant mothers are naturally concerned about the health of their babies, and modern techniques such as ultrasound help to reassure them that all is well. Other routine tests that will be needed during pregnancy include urine tests, blood samples, and regular checking of the mother's blood pressure.*

▼ *Women who are pregnant no longer feel that they must hide themselves away from the public gaze. In fact, their appearance is often enhanced by the rosy bloom of pregnancy and their own sense of well-being.*

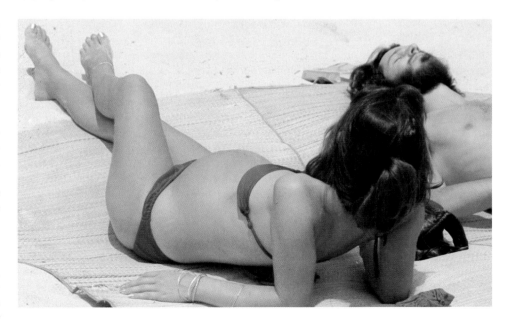

6 WEEKS

▼ *At six weeks of pregnancy the embryo is still not recognizably human, and it is only 0.5 in. (about 1.3 cm) long. A pregnancy test now would be positive, and the mother may feel some symptoms such as breast sensitivity and nausea.*

12 WEEKS

▼ *At 12 weeks the uterus can just be felt above the pelvis. By now all the major fetal organs are formed; nails are appearing on the fingers and toes. The fetus is about 3 in. (7.5 cm) long and weighs about 0.5 oz. (14 g). The mother's breasts begin to produce colostrum.*

20 WEEKS

▼ *By 20 weeks of pregnancy the uterus has reached the level of the mother's navel, and she starts to become aware of some of the movements of her baby. The fetus now measures about 8 in. (21 cm) and is covered with fine, downy hair called lanugo.*

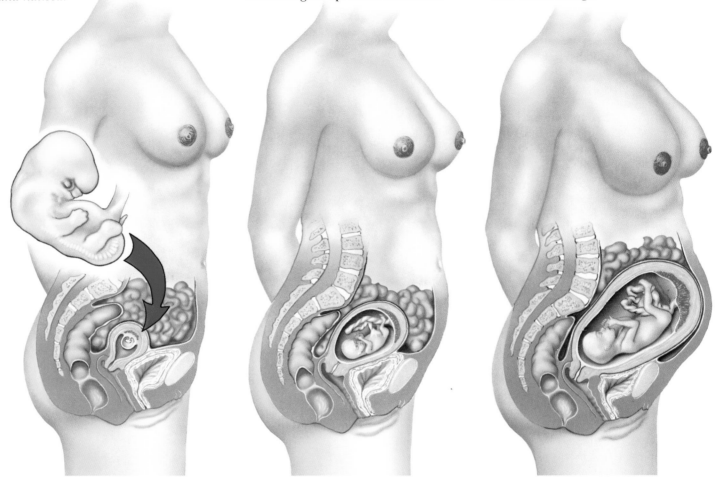

sample taken. On some visits, a blood sample will also be taken from the mother in order to establish her blood group and type, to check that she is not anemic, and to find out if there are antibodies present (see Rubella). This sample can also reveal if the placenta, through which the fetus is nourished in the uterus, is working efficiently. Some fetal abnormalities can also show up in tests of the mother's blood, although further tests would be needed to definitely confirm the presence of this abnormality in the fetus.

Every prenatal checkup includes an examination of the mother's abdomen to establish the baby's size and position. Internal examinations are usually done late in pregnancy and at the beginning of labor (see Internal Examination).

In addition to the routine checks, there are certain specialized tests which are carried out in certain cases to check the welfare of the fetus.

Amniocentesis: A sample of the amniotic fluid which surrounds the baby in the uterus may be tested if there is a risk that the baby is abnormal (see Amniocentesis). For example, women over 40 who

are pregnant for the first time are more likely to give birth to a baby with Down syndrome. An alternative to amniocentesis is a biopsy of the chorionic membranes that surround the fetus (see Chorionic Villus Sampling). Amniocentesis can detect Down syndrome, and also spina bifida and rhesus disease (see Down Syndrome; Spina Bifida). If for any reason the baby might have to be delivered early— for example, if it is not growing well—amniocentesis can reveal whether the baby's lungs are mature enough for it to survive.

Ultrasound: This form of examination, using high-frequency, inaudible sound waves, involves passing a scanner over the woman's lubricated abdomen. The uterus and its contents can then be viewed on a video display. In this way, the size of the baby, the position of the placenta, and even the presence of twins or triplets can all be established (see Ultrasound).

X rays: These are seldom used and are carried out only in late pregnancy when they are safer for the baby (see X Rays). In certain cases they are used to show whether the mother's pelvis is wide

28 WEEKS

▼ *At 28 weeks the uterus reaches about halfway between the navel and the breastbone. The fetal movements are more vigorous, and the mother may feel painless rhythmic contractions. The fetus is now viable, meaning that if it was born at this stage it could survive. Its skin is covered by a protective coating called vernix, and it can now open its eyes. It measures about 15 in. (38 cm).*

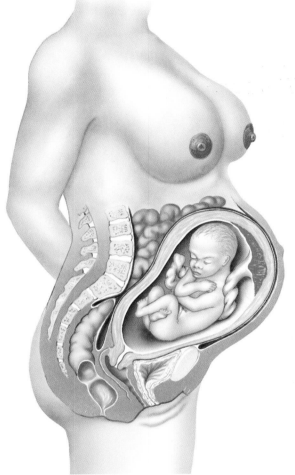

40 WEEKS

▼ *At 40 weeks the pregnancy is at full term and the mother is often impatient to get on with the delivery of her child. The upper edge of the uterus descends from its position high under the rib cage as the head of the baby moves down into the mother's pelvis. This is called engagement. The mother's breathing and digestion become easier, although pressure on her bladder increases.*

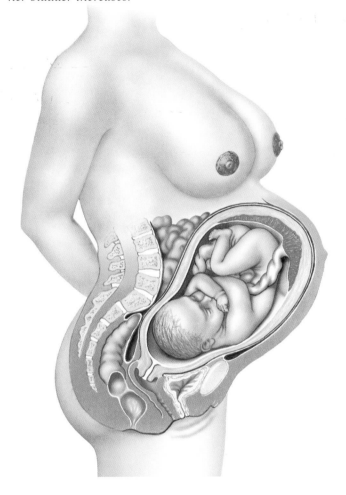

enough to allow the baby's head to pass through easily (see Pelvis), or, if not, whether delivery by cesarean section will be necessary (see Cesarean Birth).

During pregnancy

It is important for a pregnant woman to eat a well-balanced diet with plenty of protein (meat, fish, cheese, milk), fresh fruit, and vegetables (see Diet). Too many cakes and cookies should be avoided, since they can lead to excessive weight gain, which will be difficult to shed after the birth.

The amount of weight gained should not be more than 26 pounds (12 kg), but a crash diets should never be embarked upon during pregnancy, because it will deprive the baby of nourishment. If a doctor has prescribed iron tablets, they should be taken regularly.

Moderate exercise is a good idea, although pregnancy is not the time to take up a new, strenuous sport. Women will be taught exercises at prenatal classes to strengthen their back and muscles.

Smoking cigarettes should be avoided at all costs. Smoking restricts the blood vessels in the placenta, decreasing blood flow. As a result the baby gets less nourishment and oxygen. Smoking even 10 cigarettes a day significantly reduces birth weight and increases the risk of mental and physical damage to the fetus (see Smoking). No drugs should be taken without the doctor's advice. While the occasional alcoholic drink will do no harm, any heavy drinking could damage the baby's brain and also slow its growth (see Fetal Alcohol Syndrome). Apart from these sensible precautions, the expectant mother should remember that pregnancy is a normal, healthy state for most women. With adequate rest, a good diet, and moderate exercise, most women pass happily through pregnancy without serious complications.

See also: **Abortion; Birth; Breast-feeding; Conception; Fetus; Hormones; Miscarriage; Morning sickness; Obstetrics; Placenta; Prenatal care**

Premature babies

The watershed in a baby's development in the uterus is technically the 37th week of pregnancy. Infants born earlier are considered to be premature and need to be cared for scrupulously until they are less vulnerable.

Questions and Answers

My daughter was born eight weeks early and weighs 2.5 lb. (1.2 kg). Will I harm her if I touch her?

No. Stroking and touching her will comfort her and help you to get to know each other. Mothers and newborn babies form a strong bond by watching and touching each other. When a baby is very small and is surrounded by medical staff and equipment, it becomes harder for this intimate relationship to develop. To overcome this, you need to spend as much time as possible with her in the baby unit.

When can a premature baby be taken home?

There is no magic weight or size that the baby must attain. When babies are feeding well from the breast or a bottle without help and their general progress is satisfactory, they can go home. The baby's room should be kept warm for the first few weeks, but otherwise he or she is just like any other normal baby born at term.

My son was born five and a half weeks early and weighed only 4.2 lb. (1.9 kg). For nine days he was given milk via a fine tube passed through his nose into his stomach. Why was this necessary?

Babies cannot suck adequately from the breast or bottle until after about 36 weeks of pregnancy. With very premature babies this difficulty can be overcome by giving the milk directly into the stomach via a nasogastric tube.

Also, preterm babies can tolerate only a small amount of milk at a time and so need to be fed small amounts frequently. This method of feeding will also prevent hypoglycemia, in which their blood sugar becomes low. Giving the milk to your baby via a nasogastric tube was a simple and effective way of feeding him until he was able to suck on his own.

A pregnancy usually lasts 40 weeks; this is calculated from the first day of the mother's last menstrual period (see Menstruation). Most babies are born between week 39 and week 41 of the pregnancy. Babies born three or more weeks early (in other words, before the 37th week of pregnancy) are considered to be premature, or preterm. The practice nowadays, however, is to assess prematurity in terms of birth weight rather than length of gestation.

Premature babies may develop a number of problems. The smaller and more premature the baby, the more severe these problems are likely to be, although even at birth every baby is unique, and it is impossible to predict exactly what may happen in every case.

Causes of premature births

The risk factors for prematurity include maternal smoking, malnutrition, drug abuse, genital infection (especially bacterial vaginosis) and low socioeconomic status (see Drug Abuse; Malnutrition; Smoking). The uterus may have an abnormal shape, and sometimes the cervix (neck of the uterus), which should stay tightly closed during the pregnancy, is loose and may open too soon.

There are times, too, when the obstetrician may decide that, despite the risks, it will be safer to deliver the baby early. This usually happens in cases where the mother becomes seriously ill, for example, from high blood pressure or if she has had a hemorrhage; it also may occur because the baby itself is sick or in some distress.

Delivery

Most premature babies will have a normal birth. It is important for them to be delivered as gently as possible, and some obstetricians use forceps to help achieve this. If the baby is very

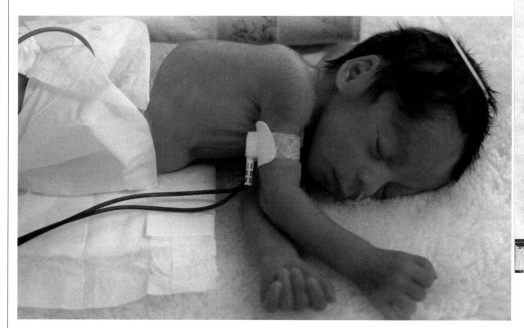

▲ *Premature babies often cannot suck well at the breast or on a bottle and have to be fed via an infusion into a vein. Babies weighing less than 4.5 lb. (2 kg) will have to be looked after in a special care baby unit, where their environment and condition can be carefully monitored by the medical staff.*

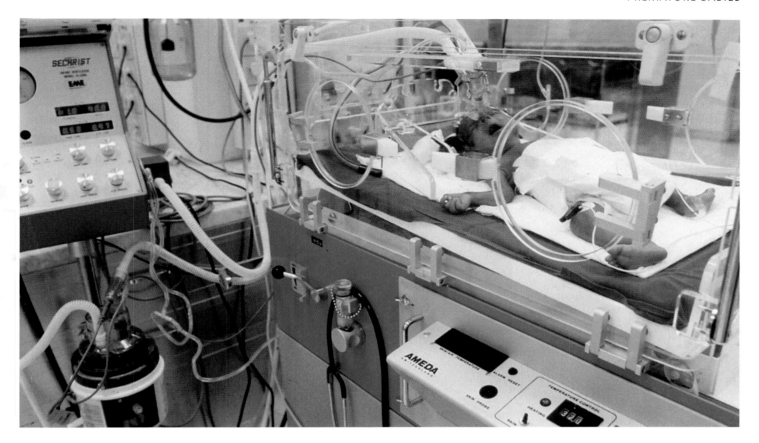

▲ *A premature baby with respiratory distress syndrome lies in an incubator in a neonatal intensive care unit surrounded by equipment to help it breathe.*

premature (more than eight weeks early), and especially if it is lying in a breech position (with the head facing up instead of down), the obstetrician will usually want to deliver the baby by cesarean section (see Cesarean Birth).

A pediatrician will always be present in case there are any complications—for example, if the baby needs help in breathing. He or she will also decide if the baby should be admitted to a special care baby unit called a neonatal intensive care unit for special attention.

Neonatal intensive care units

These units provide expert medical and nursing care for babies who are sick or small. Naturally, every mother wants to have her newborn baby with her to hold, feed, and care for. The first few days are the most important for a mother and baby to get to know each other and to develop a strong bond, so separating a mother from her baby and sending the infant to a neonatal intensive care unit is clearly undesirable. Nevertheless, this may be necessary in certain situations.

Any baby who is ill or weighs less than 4.5 pounds (2 kg) will have to be looked after in a special care baby unit. Babies just above this weight will still need special attention, which may be given in a baby unit; in some hospitals it may be given on the maternity floor. The bustle and efficiency of the medical staff, and the equipment surrounding tiny, helpless babies, can make the neonatal intensive care unit seem like an overwhelming and impersonal place. However, usually the strangeness of the unit recedes as the parents get used to it and get to know the staff and their own baby better.

The preterm baby

Preterm infants may look very frail, but they are usually very active. Even those born 12 weeks too early can open their eyes and can respond to sound, light, and touch. They will cry, of course, but usually less often and not as strongly as a baby born at term. The abdomen of a premature baby, compared with a baby born at term, is disproportionately larger, the arms and legs are skinny and wrinkled, and the skin may be covered with fine hair. Premature babies have problems feeding, keeping warm, and breathing, and with jaundice. They may also be prone to infection because, unlike babies born at term, their defenses are often not yet fully developed (see Fetus).

Warmth

Small babies need to be kept warm. The surface area of any baby's skin is very large compared with the size of the body, and premature babies are especially likely to become cold, since they lose heat far more quickly than full-term babies. A baby that is only slightly underweight but otherwise healthy may be wrapped warmly and nursed in a heated room. A baby who is smaller or needs to be kept under close observation will be nursed in an incubator.

Feeding

Special feeding techniques are often needed for preterm babies because they usually cannot suck at the breast or on a bottle (see Breast-Feeding). In such cases, milk may be fed directly into the stomach through a fine tube. Gradually, as the baby learns to suck and becomes stronger, he or she will be able to adjust to the mother's breast or to a bottle. Occasionally, it may be necessary to provide all the baby's nutrition via an IV infusion into a vein (see Intravenous Infusion), then gradually introduce milk when he or she can tolerate it.

It is very important to me that I breast-feed my baby. If he or she is born prematurely, is breast-feeding still possible?

Yes, it is still possible to give breast milk to even very tiny babies. One of the advantages of breast milk is that it will help protect your baby from infections. If your baby is too young to suck at the breast, the milk can be expressed (squeezed out). This can be made easier with the help of a breast pump and can be done either at the hospital or at home; the milk is frozen and used as required. The milk can be given via a nasogastric tube until your baby is old enough to start feeding from the breast. Many mothers supply special care baby units with extra breast milk, and this can be used to feed some of the other premature babies.

I remained very active until late in my pregnancy, but my baby was born four weeks early. I cannot relate it to anything I did, but could it have been my fault?

It was not your fault that you went into labor early. Occasionally women blame a very bad fall or a severe emotional upset, but it is actually extremely uncommon for there to have been any untoward incident shortly before the onset of labor. In most instances it is unknown why labor should start early. There are sometimes medical causes, and you should ask your obstetrician about them before you leave the hospital.

Why do very premature babies have to be put in incubators?

A very premature baby can survive outside the womb, but the chances of remaining healthy are better if he or she initially stays in the stable, germ-free environment an incubator provides. An incubator is a flat cradle with a transparent cover in which the air is kept at the correct temperature and humidity. The mother should spend as much time as possible in the same room as the incubator to develop the bond between her and her child.

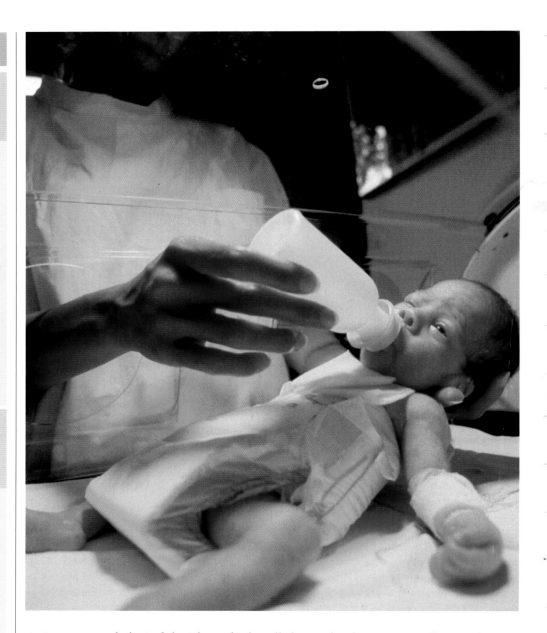

▲ *A premature baby is fed with mother's milk from a bottle. Human milk provides valuable antibodies to help the baby fight infections.*

Breathing problems

The premature baby, especially one born very early, is prone to having breathing problems (see Breathing). The pattern of breathing will not be as regular as that of a more mature baby. Sometimes these irregularities become very pronounced and the baby may not breathe for several seconds. The preterm baby will actually outgrow these prolonged pauses in breathing (called apneic episodes) in time, but until then he or she must be observed very carefully.

Babies who have difficulty breathing may be nursed on a special apnea mattress, and the rate of their breathing and heartbeat may be monitored by leads attached to the baby's chest. If the apneic episodes are short and not too frequent, they can be terminated by a little gentle stimulation, which reminds the baby to breathe. If the episodes are prolonged and frequent, the baby may need a respirator to assist with breathing (see Respirators).

Another breathing problem from which premature babies may suffer is shortage of oxygen due to respiratory distress syndrome. Some babies are born before the membrane that lines the inside of the lungs has developed, and they become short of oxygen because they cannot expand their lungs properly (see Lung and Lung Diseases). The mature lung produces a substance called surfactant that makes the lungs easy to inflate. A surfactant is a detergent-like substance that

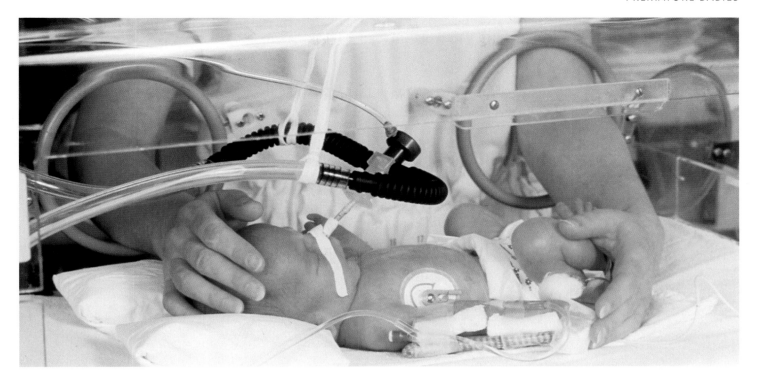

▲ *Neonatal intensive care units are beehives of activity. To the mother, her baby may initially seem hedged in by doctors, nurses, and sophisticated equipment—on the surface, not the best atmosphere for developing the essential bond between mother and child. However, the mother can spend all the time she wants getting to know her baby in the unit. She will be able to cuddle the baby, see the nurses tending him or her, or simply keep watch beside the incubator.*

markedly reduces surface tension so that wet surfaces that are in contact with each other can separate more easily. Surfactant is not produced normally in some premature babies, and this makes it very difficult to inflate the lungs and supply oxygen to the body.

If the correct amount of oxygen and support for the baby's breathing can be provided, the membrane will usually be formed by around the tenth day and the lungs will be normal from then onward. Artificial surfactant may be helpful in the meantime.

Jaundice

Jaundice is a very common problem in premature babies. It occurs when a yellow pigment, called bilirubin, accumulates in the blood and skin, causing discoloration. This may be because the liver, which breaks down the bilirubin, is not mature enough to cope immediately (see Liver and Liver Diseases). Usually the jaundice is mild and harmless and fades away within a week or so of birth.

Sometimes, however, the jaundice in a premature baby can become more marked and presents a serious problem. If the level of bilirubin in the bloodstream becomes too high, it can damage the baby's hearing and the developing brain. However, jaundice can be treated using phototherapy; this involves placing the baby under a bank of blue fluorescent lights, which convert the bilirubin in the blood and skin to a water-soluble form that can be excreted in the urine. Exchange blood transfusions are also used in extreme cases of jaundice (see Blood Transfusion).

The infant with very low birthweight

Most premature babies are born only a few weeks early. They may need help with feeding and keeping warm, and they may occasionally experience other, more serious problems, but with the facilities available in neonatal intensive care units the outlook for them is now excellent. However, the infant with very low birthweight, who weighs less than 3.7 pounds (1.5 kg) and was born more than eight weeks early, is likely to suffer many more problems and will need the expert facilities of an intensive care unit. It is impossible to provide such specialized facilities in every hospital, so these units are usually centralized, with one or two in an area. The mother can sometimes be transferred to a hospital with the necessary care facilities before the birth if it is anticipated that her baby is going to be very preterm; alternatively, the baby will be transferred directly after birth. A very ill baby or one requiring surgery would also need to be transferred to a neonatal intensive care unit.

Leaving the hospital

As the premature baby gets older and begins to put on weight, the parents can take over from the nurses and hold, cuddle, feed, and play with their baby. When the time approaches for the baby to go home, facilities are usually made available for the mother to come back into the hospital and have the opportunity of taking care of her baby entirely on her own for a few days before the baby leaves the unit. This will allow the mother to gain confidence in her ability to look after her baby (particularly if it is her first), and it also gives the mother the chance to get to know her baby, and to feel that he or she truly belongs to her. Once the premature baby leaves the unit and goes home, he or she can, and should, be treated like any other baby.

See also: **Birth; Breech birth; Cervix and cervical smears; Child development; Jaundice; Neonatal intensive care unit; Obstetrics; Oxygen; Pediatric medicine; Pregnancy; Uterus**

Premedication

Questions and Answers

Does premedication affect people in different ways?

Yes. The amount of drug that is given is estimated according to the size of the patient, but sensitivity can vary. Some patients notice a marked effect, while others feel no effect at all. Generally, a patient who has been taking medicines at home, for instance for pain, or a patient who has been drinking heavily over a long period, might find premedication less effective. Other patients fall into a deep sleep after only a small dose.

I am afraid of injections. Can a premed be given any other way?

Yes, though the drugs used in premedication usually do have to be injected. The anesthesiologist who orders the drug may suggest giving a patient a tablet of a substance such as diazepam (Valium) with a little water. Then once the patient has been anesthetized, he or she can be injected with the other drugs.

Will I do anything embarrassing under the influence of a premed?

Possibly. The drugs that are used can sometimes have an effect on inhibitions. You may feel so relaxed and unconcerned that you become very talkative and giggly. This sort of thing does not occur very often, though. The patient usually just becomes very sleepy.

Is it possible to be allergic to premeds in the same way that, say, you can be allergic to penicillin?

Yes, but such an allergy is very rare. Atropine, a drug used to dry up the secretions in the mouth and throat, can cause a rash on the neck and chest, but this usually goes away after a few hours. Allergies to opiate drugs are possible but are also very rare.

Most of the people who go into the hospital for surgery are given premedication (also called a "premed") to relax them just before they are taken to the operating room. Why is this necessary?

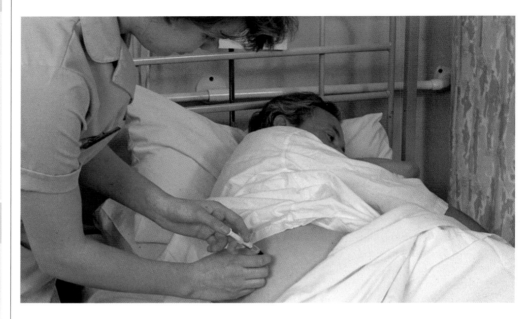

▲ *Premedication is injected before surgery to calm the patient and decrease the secretions produced by the air passages and salivary glands, thus making the anesthetist's job easier.*

Premedication is given to patients just before surgery or before other investigations, such as special X rays, that may require anesthesia (see X Rays). There are three main purposes for premedication: to allay anxiety in patients who are likely to be nervous and frightened before a surgical procedure; to decrease the secretions normally produced by the lining of the air passages and the salivary glands, making the anesthetist's job easier and safer; and to decrease the amount of anesthesia needed during the first part of an operation, since a painkilling drug has already been given.

The drugs used and their dangers

Two main groups of drugs are used in premedication. The first are opiate drugs such as fentanyl that are chemically related to morphine. These drugs act on the central nervous system, suppressing the awareness of pain. At the same time, they make patients feel calm and relaxed.

The second group includes compounds such as atropine and scopolamine; these are similar to the substance found in the plant deadly nightshade. These drugs act in the periphery of the body at certain nerve endings, and cause a decrease in the activity of the tiny glands that line the mouth and air passages, as well as the salivary glands. Before these drugs were used routinely, patients produced large amounts of watery fluid in their mouths and airways in response to the irritant effects of the anesthetics being inhaled. This could cause serious problems by obstructing the airways and lead to suffocation. Other sedative drugs used as premedication include diazepam (Valium) and promazine (Sparine). Premedication drugs are usually given by an intramuscular injection about an hour before surgery. They can sometimes have undesirable side effects. Some patients on an opiate drug may hallucinate. Atropine and its related compounds can cause an uncomfortably dry mouth and, in some cases, a bright red rash on the neck and chest, though this will disappear within a few hours.

See also: Anesthetics; Injections; Morphine; Painkillers; Sedatives; Side effects; Surgery

Premenstrual syndrome

Questions and Answers

I have never suffered from premenstrual syndrome (PMS) but my mother told me that I might develop it after I have had a baby, since this happened to her. I am pregnant at the moment and am worried that PMS will start after the baby is born. If my mother is right, is there anything I can do to make sure it doesn't happen?

Some women find that PMS does not occur until after the birth of their first baby. It is hard to know whether this will happen to you, but it is important not to worry about it, or you'll find yourself looking for symptoms, which may make you feel tense and anxious.

My 15-year-old daughter becomes impossible to live with immediately before her period. She's very grumpy and bad-tempered, and as a result we are always arguing. What can I do to help her?

Start by discussing what you have noticed and see if she has noticed a pattern of negative feelings that immediately precede her periods. If she has, you may find that your doctor can help. You should try to avoid getting into arguments with her, which will make both of you feel angry and depressed. She may find it useful to read a book about premenstrual syndrome so that she can understand what is happening to her; this may make it easier for her to cope with it.

I went to see my doctor about my PMS but he just told me to get more sleep and exercise. I've tried this and it hasn't helped. My friend told me that PMS can be treated, so what should I do now?

Go back to your doctor and tell him that his suggestions have not helped. He may then be able to refer you to a specialist or a clinic for investigation and treatment. If he refuses to help, it might be useful to see another doctor.

Premenstrual syndrome, or PMS, can make a woman's life a misery before menstruation. Medical treatment can relieve some symptoms, but self-help and understanding from friends can also alleviate much of the distress.

Not every woman going through the menstrual cycle has problems in the premenstrual phase. While some women experience changes in their body, or moods, they do not find these distressing enough to seek treatment; others even report feeling particularly productive and fit during the premenstrual phase. However, over 50 percent of women are thought to suffer from noticeable premenstrual symptoms, and about 10 percent of these need treatment.

The menstrual cycle

If a woman regularly experiences premenstrual syndrome, commonly called PMS, or suspects that she might, it is important for her to understand what happens during the menstrual cycle. The average premenstrual cycle is 28 days (see diagram on page 1673), but the length varies from woman to woman and may be longer or shorter.

During menstruation the uterine lining is shed and the body gets ready to begin a new cycle. The period lasts for about five days, and as soon as menstruation stops, the pituitary gland in the brain sends a hormonal message to one of the two ovaries, telling it to mature an egg follicle (see Ovaries; Pituitary Gland).

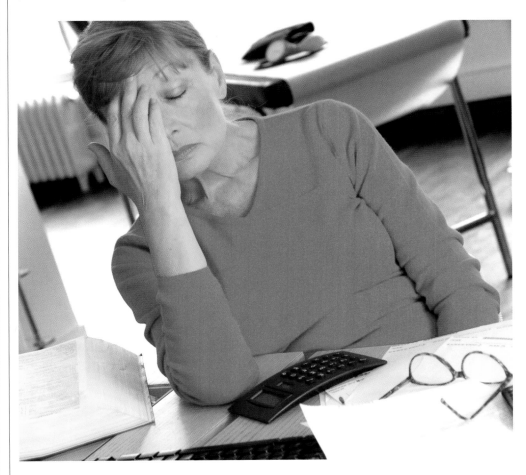

▲ *A woman who suffers from migraines will find she is more prone to migraine attacks when she is premenstrual. PMS symptoms can greatly interfere with her work.*

Questions and Answers

I'm sure that I get PMS, but my husband says that it's just psychosomatic and that I'm making a fuss about nothing. Is it possible that he could be right and that I am just imagining it?

It can be very upsetting to be told that there is nothing wrong with you when you are sure there is. If you have discovered a clear relationship between how you feel and your menstrual cycle then it is likely that you do get PMS. Your husband should try to accept this and be more supportive. His lack of sympathy may make your tension worse, and you should make this clear to him if it is so. If you can see your doctor and get his or her help, this might convince your husband that you do get PMS. No one knows what role social and psychological factors have in causing premenstrual syndrome, but it is clear that it is a real, severe problem for many women.

I am on a diet at the moment and get really disheartened when my weight goes up before a period. Should I restrict my eating even more during this time?

No. The weight gain is almost certainly due to water retention, and will disappear once your period has begun. You should eat sensibly throughout the premenstruum and cut your fluid intake to about four cups a day. You should also reduce the amount of salt in your diet, because salt increases water retention. Don't go without food for hours at a time, since this may result in your feeling faint and dizzy. Experts on the premenstrual phase say that you should eat little but often during the days before a period.

Will I stop suffering from PMS once I have reached menopause?

At menopause you no longer go through the menstrual cycle; thus you will no longer get PMS. Any depression, anxiety, or mood swings may be due to other hormonal cycles, which your doctor may be able to help you with.

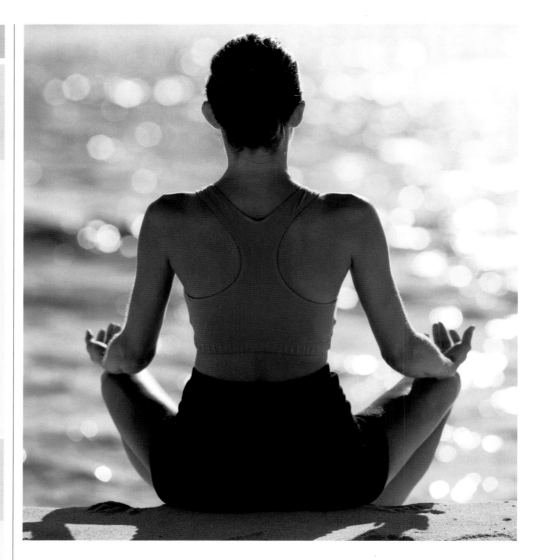

▲ *Women who suffer from physical or emotional tension before their menstrual periods may benefit from yoga or similar exercise that helps relax both the body and the mind.*

The hormone estrogen is then produced from the graafian follicle (made up of the egg and the cells surrounding it); one of the functions of estrogen is to begin preparation of the lining of the uterus for a possible pregnancy (see Uterus). The amount of estrogen that is produced continues to rise until it is time for ovulation (see Estrogen).

Around the 14th day of the cycle the egg is fully ripened. The pituitary gland then releases another hormone to stimulate the release of the egg, which travels into the fallopian tube adjacent to the ovary. The follicle left behind after ovulation now starts to produce the hormones estrogen and progesterone, which make the uterine lining thicker and spongier, ready to nourish a fertilized egg. At this stage of the cycle a pregnancy can occur, but this is possible for only a day or so.

If the egg is not fertilized, it quickly begins to degenerate. The levels of estrogen and progesterone begin to fall, and, as a result, the uterine lining cannot be maintained. The lining is then shed, and the cycle begins again. It is during the second phase of the menstrual cycle that women who suffer from PMS may experience symptoms.

Symptoms and related problems

Physical symptoms of the premenstruum (the days immediately preceding menstruation) vary widely in type and severity from woman to woman. For example, one woman experiences slight tenderness and swelling of the breasts while another experiences swelling in most parts of her body, making her feel clumsy and awkward. Swelling and bloatedness are related to water retention. Not all water taken into the body is passed in urine; some accumulates in body cells and tissues, causing weight gain in some women, who put on 3 to 6.5 pounds (1.5–3 kg) just before menstruation.

Other physical symptoms associated with PMS are skin problems such as pimples or blotchiness, an increase in the likelihood of cystitis, and a general feeling of being under the weather (see Cystitis). Women who suffer from conditions such as epilepsy, asthma, migraine, and conjunctivitis may find that their conditions worsen at this time. Some women even find that their contact lenses become uncomfortable.

The reasons for these symptoms are not yet fully understood. What is known is that the symptoms are likely to improve once menstruation begins and return at the next premenstrual phase.

The psychological symptoms that are related to PMS are also likely to improve as soon as the period starts. A woman with PMS may feel depressed and anxious in the days before her period, suffer from lack of energy and a marked increase in irritability, be less interested in sex, or find it difficult to concentrate. Because any one of these problems can exist independently of the premenstruum, it can be difficult to diagnose PMS.

A number of research studies have suggested that women are more likely to commit crimes and acts of aggression during the premenstrual phase and that they are most likely to attempt suicide in the days before a period (see Suicide).

PMS is also said to cause marital problems and in some cases to lead to divorce; however, it is just as likely that marital problems can increase the likelihood of PMS.

Causes

Although a number of explanations have been put forward, scientific debate is still going on about the causes of PMS. Some doctors believe it is directly related to problems with the production and balance of progesterone and estrogen in the body. Others suggest that the brain may not be producing the correct amount of a chemical called pyridoxine.

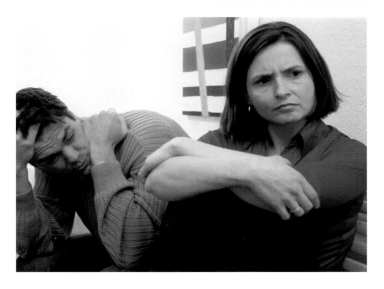

▲ *Symptoms of PMS such as aggression, irritability, and depression can lead to arguments and marital problems. Alternatively, marital problems can increase symptoms of PMS.*

However, nonmedical factors could also be partly responsible for PMS. It may be that many women are ashamed of their body's reproductive processes or associate the menstrual cycle with something negative. Because it is difficult to measure the effect of such ideas on individual women, it is also difficult to arrive at any proof for such theories.

Diagnosing the problem

Any problems that occur particularly during the premenstruum may be a sign that a woman suffers from PMS. She may find that her mood swings and physical symptoms follow a pattern coinciding

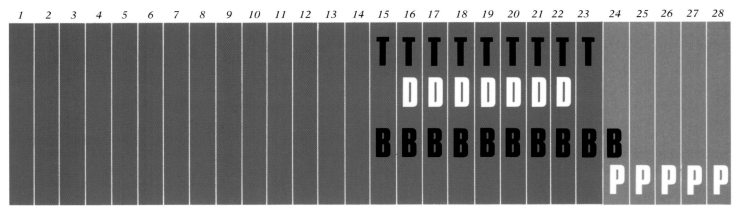

CHARTING SYMPTOMS OF PMS

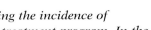

▲ *A woman who suspects that she suffers from PMS should keep a calendar of her symptoms, noting the incidence of headaches, back pain, tension and so on. This will help her and her gynecologist to plan a suitable treatment program. In the above example, day 1 of the menstrual cycle is taken as the day after the end of menstruation.*

with the days before menstruation. One way to discover if this is the case is to record the changes in a diary, calendar, or chart. As a result, a woman may discover that she is especially clumsy, quick-tempered, or tired in the days just before her period, and the record will also be useful for her gynecologist if she decides to seek medical help.

She should keep a record for at least three months; if she finds a clear pattern of negative symptoms, she may be able to help herself.

Self-help

A woman should try to adjust her routine in the days before a period so that she does not put herself under physical stress. This applies particularly to dieting, which may increase the likelihood of faintness or dizziness. She should avoid strict dieting during the premenstrual phase and make certain that she eats regularly, little but often, when premenstrual problems arise.

Some experts recommend reducing liquid intake to about four cups a day if a woman suffers from water retention. A reduction in salt in the diet may also help, since salt increases water retention (see Salt).

Exercise can also help a woman with PMS a great deal and will make her feel generally fitter (see Exercise). Relaxation exercises can help with tension, both physical and emotional (see Relaxation).

If a woman finds that premenstrual problems affect her emotions—if she feels irritable or depressed, for example—it is important for her to explain to those close to her what is happening. She may wish to warn them that her reactions to difficulties are likely to be more intense during this time, and to ask for their understanding and support. It is impossible to avoid all problems during this phase, but planning may enable her to avoid particularly stressful occasions and obligations (see Stress). However, there is no reason for PMS to prevent her from doing things that she wishes to do.

Help from the doctor

Various types of medication can help relieve PMS, but currently there is no one solution that is helpful to all women.

Most doctors prescribe one of two types of treatment: hormone tablets or vitamin B6. Progesterone therapy is based on the theory that PMS is caused by a lack of progesterone and can therefore be cured by improving the hormone balance. A woman with PMS will be given tablets, suppositories, or a shot (see Injections; Suppositories). The amount and frequency of treatment will depend on her symptoms, the type of progesterone used, and how successful the therapy is in her case. The dosage may be increased if her symptoms do not improve after a time.

Some doctors prescribe an oral contraceptive to help a woman with PMS, but this may not be suitable for her and may not even work if it is suitable. The Pill prevents a normal menstrual cycle from taking place, but is unlikely to have any lasting effect after a woman stops taking it. Some women find that they have PMS just as severely on the Pill as they do ordinarily.

Some studies have indicated that vitamin B6—a coenzyme that is involved in amino acid metabolism and essential for the formation of new amino acid in many of the body's metabolic processes—may be effective in reducing the symptoms of PMS. It can be prescribed by a doctor or bought from a drugstore. Tablets are taken from three days before symptoms are expected until the period starts. The initial dose may be 2 mg twice a day, but may be increased if there is no effect. If a woman buys the vitamin over the counter at a drugstore, she should

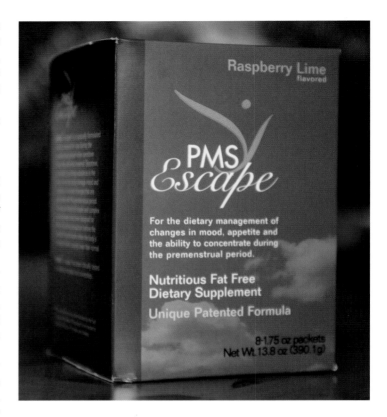

▲ *Some products are available to help women manage PMS. Studies of* **PMS Escape**—*which contains vitamin C, vitamin B6, magnesium, calcium, and carbohydrates—indicate that it can reduce cravings for sweet and starchy carbohydrates and improve moods, reducing anger and irritability, by boosting levels of serotonin (the brain's natural mood manager) that are deficient in women during the premenstruum.*

ask her doctor about dosage and any changes to her diet while she is taking it. Vitamin B6 can cause nerve damage if taken in excess, so the dosage should be monitored by a doctor. Some doctors believe that dosages over 20 mg may cause a risk of nerve damage. The vitamin is intended to replace the brain chemical pyridoxine. The benefits may take a month or two to be noticed, but many women report that vitamin B6 has put an end to monthly problems such as depression, anxiety, and headaches.

Tranquilizers and antidepressants may be prescribed for a woman with PMS if her doctor is unsure whether or not her problems are caused by PMS. However, many women find that these drugs create new problems such as lethargy and lack of concentration and are therefore of no help (see Tranquilizers).

In the past, diuretics were used to reduce water retention during the premenstrual phase. However, they should not be bought over the counter at a drugstore and should be taken only if prescribed by a doctor. Taking too high a dose of diuretics can cause other medical problems. Cutting down fluid intake and salt may be a more useful way of helping to reduce water retention.

See also: **Breasts; Diuretics; Gynecology; Headache; Hormones; Lethargy; Menstruation; Oral contraceptives; Skin and skin diseases; Vitamin B**

Prenatal care

Years ago I thought I had a sexually transmitted disease but never went for a checkup. Now I am pregnant. Could I pass it on to my baby?

Discuss your concerns with your obstetrician. Some STDs, such as syphilis, are passed on to the baby in the uterus, and may cause birth defects. Others, like gonorrhea, are passed on at the time of birth, and may require special treatment to protect the baby's eyes.

Someone told me that scrubbing my nipples with a nailbrush will prepare them for breast-feeding. Is this really necessary?

Certainly not. You need only moisturize your breasts in the same way as the rest of your body, and wear a good bra. If you have inturned nipples (nipples that do not stick out), ask your doctor for advice, since there could be problems with breast-feeding.

Is it possible to know the sex of my baby before it is born? If so, how?

A test called amniocentesis, carried out to screen for genetic disorders, can show the baby's sex. However, it carries a small risk and is not performed just to identify sex. Later in the pregnancy the gender is visible on ultrasound scanning.

I am in my eighth month of pregnancy. Is it dangerous for my partner and me to make love?

If you and the baby are in good health, there is no reason why you should not continue making love with your partner to the end of your pregnancy—it is probably very good for your relationship. If you have problems finding a comfortable position, try something new—ideally where penetration is not too deep. Should there be any discomfort, pain, or bleeding, see your doctor at once.

For an expectant mother, it is vitally important to stay fit and well throughout her pregnancy. Proper prenatal care will help ensure that she achieves an easy birth and a healthy baby.

The likelihood of a child's dying before one year of age is doubled if the mother has had no prenatal care prior to the birth. Care for both mother and baby during pregnancy should involve regular visits to the obstetrician, a balanced diet, and controlled daily exercise and rest in preparation for the exertions of the labor itself.

Diet and general health

It is essential to maintain a well-balanced diet during pregnancy. However, a pregnant woman does not need to eat for two. Gaining too much weight is bad for both mother and baby and makes it more difficult for the mother to get her figure back after the birth. The total weight gain during pregnancy should not be more than 25 to 28 pounds (12–14 kg). It is important for a pregnant woman to ensure that she gets the best nutritional value from her food and eats sensible quantities (see Diet; Nutrition).

The daily diet of a pregnant woman should include protein. This can be obtained in two or three helpings of meat, fish, or cheese; 1 pint (0.5 l) of milk; two helpings of vegetables and salad; two portions of fresh fruit, including one citrus fruit or its juice; butter or margarine in

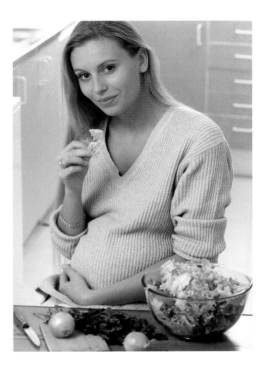

▲ *Pregnant women are advised to eat two helpings of salad a day. Green leafy vegetables contain folic acid, which helps prevent neural tube defects in the fetus.*

moderation; and four to five slices of whole-grain bread (or cereal or pasta instead of bread). Vitamins also play an important part in general health and are easily obtained through a sensible, well-balanced diet. Routine multivitamin supplements during pregnancy are not needed, unless the doctor advises otherwise. However, folic acid may prevent some birth defects (see Vitamin B). Minerals are as important as vitamins and are also available in normal foods (see Minerals). Some obstetricians recommend that expectant mothers take iron tablets as a routine measure during the last three months of pregnancy, and calcium is also often given as a supplement (see Calcium; Iron).

Self-help

Though pregnancy is certainly not a disease, many women suffer from a variety of minor ailments, which make them miserable. Most of these can be avoided or alleviated with a little care.

Women suffering from nausea and vomiting should eat a dry cookie with a cup of tea before getting up in the morning. It helps to eat frequent small meals. To prevent indigestion and heartburn, pregnant women should avoid fried foods and late meals, and allow plenty of time to digest food before going to bed. They can avoid constipation and hemorrhoids by including roughage in the diet: vegetables, fruit, whole-grain bread, bran, and cereal (see Constipation; Hemorrhoids). They should also drink about six to eight glasses of water every day and take plenty of gentle exercise, such as walking or yoga. Backache can be a problem, so pregnant women should pay attention to their posture, and avoid picking up or carrying heavy items (see Back and

I am a twin and my husband's family also has a history of twins. I am now 12 weeks' pregnant. How soon can I find out whether I am going to have one child or more?

Sixteen weeks is the earliest that you can be sure of clear results from an ultrasound scan, which many obstetricians run as a matter of routine at this stage. In view of the history of twins, your obstetrician will be on the alert for them in your case.

I have a very small frame and my baby is thought to be very large. My doctor wants me to have an X ray to see the size of the baby's head in relation to my pelvis. Will this damage my unborn child?

The doctor will not take the X ray until the last four weeks of pregnancy. The fetus is most vulnerable to damage by the rays in its first three months. This applies to X rays on any part of the body, so remember to tell the dentist that you are pregnant if he or she wants to X-ray your teeth. X rays are hardly ever used on expectant mothers these days; ultrasound is considered sufficient in most cases. However, there are exceptions, such as when there is doubt about the size of the pelvis, the baby is incorrectly positioned, or the baby is upside down and a breech birth is expected.

My husband and I both feel that he should attend our baby's birth. Is this really a good thing?

Most hospitals welcome the presence of the father at the birth, to reassure the mother and share in the experience. Many prenatal classes also involve the father, preparing him to help during the labor rather than just watch. The obstetrician may allow your husband to help you give birth by holding up your legs and putting an arm around you to support your back. He can also guide you through your contractions if you are using relaxation techniques. You can both benefit from sharing the moments following the birth.

Backache). To prevent varicose veins from getting worse, they should wear support hose and avoid standing still for too long at a time: walking around is better exercise and improves the circulation. It is good to prop up the feet if possible (see Varicose Veins). Pregnant women should care for their teeth and spend time on dental hygiene daily. They should floss, massage their gums, and avoid sweet foods (see Dental Care). Finally, they should guard against any risk to the developing fetus by limiting their intake of alcohol and by not smoking (see Fetal Alcohol Syndrome; Smoking)—both alcohol and smoking are potentially harmful. Women who take any medications should ask their doctor if these are safe.

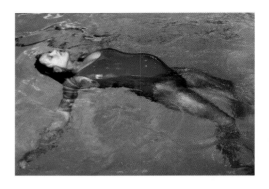

▲ *Deep relaxation is important during pregnancy. It can be practiced by floating on the back in water, or lying in bed and allowing the body to entirely let go.*

Medical care

As soon as the pregnancy has been confirmed, the obstetrician will discuss the woman's arrangements for medical care during the pregnancy, and will also arrange for the woman to go for delivery to the hospital where he or she has admitting rights.

Throughout the pregnancy the woman should make regular visits to her obstetrician's office, where a variety of tests will be carried out, and she can discuss any concerns.

These visits will probably be on a monthly basis throughout the first 28 weeks of pregnancy, then every two weeks until 36 weeks, and weekly from then on until the baby is actually born. This is only a guide, though; the schedule of visits can be flexible to allow for any unusual circumstances.

Tests you may be given

TEST	HOW OFTEN	REASON
Urine	Each prenatal visit; occasionally a 24-hour sample is collected	To check sugar and protein levels; to check hormone levels to see if the placenta, which links the mother and baby, is functioning correctly
Cervical smear	Once	Cells are analyzed to see whether there are any infections, such as gonorrhea or yeast, or early precancerous changes
Blood tests	First prenatal test	Blood group is established and checked for: antibodies that could affect the baby; hemoglobin level for anemia; STD; susceptibility to German measles
	16–17 weeks	Defects in baby, such as anencephaly; other defects in the neural tube (the tube from which the nervous system develops)
	Subsequent	Anemia, if condition is suspected on first visit
Ultrasound scan	At 16 weeks	Establishes size of baby; measures fetal heartbeat. Ultrasound is a way of monitoring a baby's development and can confirm the number of babies in the uterus.
Amniocentesis	Once, if mother is over 35 or if there is a possibility of a genetic abnormality	To perform genetic analysis for Down syndrome, spina bifida, or other neural tube defects

Exercise and posture during pregnancy

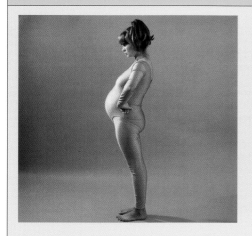

▲ Incorrect standing posture: avoid the natural tendency to compensate for the extra weight by leaning backward.

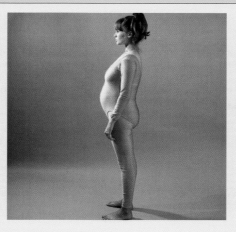

▲ Correct standing posture: stand straight with shoulders relaxed and abdomen and bottom tucked in.

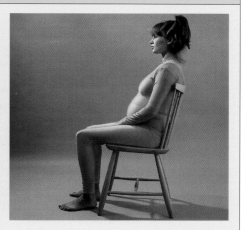

▲ Sit comfortably, in a relaxed position, with your back straight and supported by the back of the hard chair.

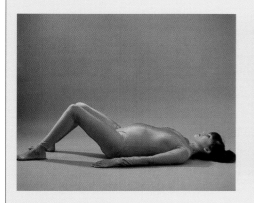

▲ For abdominal muscle tone; lie on floor as shown, tighten abdomen, pulling baby toward the backbone.

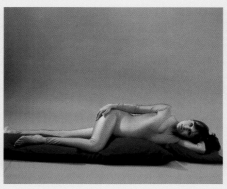

▲ In late pregnancy many women prefer to sleep on their side. A cushion between the legs gives extra comfort.

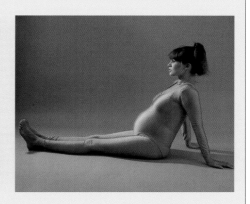

▲ In this position, practice tensing and relaxing the muscles around the anus and around the vagina and urethra.

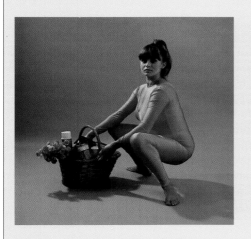

▲ In lifting an object, keep the back straight and bend from the knees. Avoid bending over, which strains muscles.

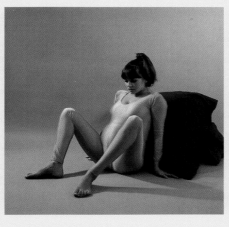

▲ Assume delivery position, as shown, with back at a 45° angle. Tense and relax pelvic floor and thigh muscles.

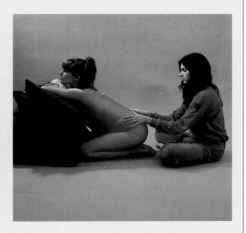

▲ Back massage will help during labor, relieving backache and contractions if they are felt in the back.

Your nutritional needs during pregnancy

NUTRIENTS	SOURCES	EFFECTS
Proteins	Meat, fish, poultry, dairy products, dried beans, peas, lentils, nuts, grains, and some vegetables	Build the tissues that form the baby, aid the growth of the placenta, and help strengthen the uterus
Carbohydrates	Flour, cereals, fruit, starchy vegetables, honey, and milk	Energy-producing foods which, if taken in excess, cause obesity. Most women, however, need more calories than usual during pregnancy.
Fats	Meat, poultry, oily fish, dairy products, eggs, oils, and nuts	Fats are necessary to a balanced diet because they help the body absorb vitamins. However, they can easily cause obesity.
Vitamin A	Dairy products, fish liver oils, margarine, oily fish, variety of meats, carrots, apricots, tomatoes, green vegetables	Good for the skin, eyes, bones, and many of the internal organs
Vitamin B group	Green leafy vegetables, whole wheat products, liver, kidneys	Counter constipation, nervousness, and skin problems; increase energy; and help form red blood cells. Folic acid may prevent neural tube defects.
Vitamin C	Citrus fruits, berry fruits, green vegetables, salad vegetables, peppers, parsley, tomatoes, and potatoes (but overcooking destroys the vitamins)	Strengthens the placenta, aids the absorption of iron, and helps in the formation of the baby's skin, hair, ligaments, and bones
Vitamin D	Fish liver oils, dairy products, oily fish, margarine, eggs, butter, cheese, liver	Helps the body absorb calcium, which is essential to build and strengthen bones
Vitamin E	Apples, carrots, cabbage, celery, eggs, muesli, olive oil, and sunflower seeds	Useful antioxidant
Vitamin K	Green leafy vegetables, eggs, cereals, potatoes, strawberries	Important in the development of the blood clotting process
Calcium	Dairy products, fish, nuts, oranges, raspberries, dried fruit, leafy green vegetables, turnips, cauliflower, and sesame seeds	Builds the bones and teeth of the growing baby
Iron	Meat (especially liver, kidney), cereal products, eggs, sardines, spinach, parsley, watercress, cocoa, chocolate, molasses, and nuts	Prevents anemia—the baby has to store a reserve of iron in its liver on which to draw while on a milk diet after birth. It saps the mother's natural supply in the womb, making supplements necessary.

Each time that the expectant mother visits the office she will be asked to provide a sample for a urine test. Her blood pressure and weight will be checked and her abdomen will be examined (see Blood Pressure). The obstetrician will listen to the fetal heartbeat, and she may have an internal examination, although this is usually done only late in the pregnancy or at the onset of labor (see Internal Examination).

Psychological preparations

During these visits to the obstetrician, the expectant mother will, of course, also be asked how she feels. There will be discussions about the emotional and physical problems that occur in pregnancy, and the reactions that may be experienced after the birth itself.

Advice on breast-feeding or bottle-feeding will be given (see Breast-Feeding). She will also be shown exercises to help her restore her figure after her baby is born. A new baby will change the lifestyle of the whole family, so expectant fathers are usually welcomed if they wish to come along on one or more visits. They can then be taught about pregnancy and labor, and will be advised about what they can do to help their partners at each stage. This will be particularly helpful in making the father feel involved, rather than rejected, after the baby is born.

Physical preparations

One of the most common problems experienced during pregnancy is bad posture, because the mother tends to overcompensate for all the extra weight that she is carrying. Expectant mothers should therefore try standing, walking, and sitting properly; good posture will soon come naturally (see Posture).

General exercises

The three main exercises to practice regularly are the pelvic floor and abdominal exercises and the birth position. There are also various relaxation techniques that can be perfected. Conscious relaxation can be practiced at any time; women should check that their facial

Yoga exercises

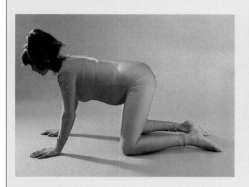

▲ *All-fours position: sit on your heels; bend forward onto knees, hands on floor; keep back straight and relaxed.*

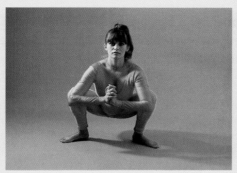

▲ *Squatting: start in a standing position, legs apart, then squat. This helps prevent backache and constipation.*

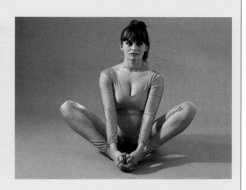

▲ *The tailor: sit upright on front of buttocks. Gently push knees down with elbows; lift thighs and lower them.*

muscles, shoulders, and hands are not tense. They should drop their shoulders and unclench their hands. Disassociation relaxation is a very good technique to learn for coping with the stresses of labor. It involves tensing one set of muscles while keeping the remaining muscles in the body relaxed. Deep relaxation is best practiced just before going to sleep by lying down and allowing the body to really let go (see Relaxation).

Breathing exercises

There are three basic breathing levels that women can use during labor. The principle in all three is always to avoid holding the breath while pushing, and to go with the contractions.

The first level can be used throughout labor, but it is especially good in the early stages. It involves deep abdominal breathing, breathing in deeply, using the abdomen on exhalation.

The second and third breathing levels are generally used as the contractions start to grow stronger. For second-level breathing, the woman should take a shallower breath and place the emphasis on the exhalation. For the third level, she should breathe in and out very gently, again placing the emphasis on exhaling.

Huffing and puffing are useful in the stage of labor just before the cervix (neck of the womb) is fully dilated. This exercise involves taking two shallow breaths while still emphasizing the exhalation each time, then blowing out quickly twice. The breath should be allowed to flow back into the lungs each time.

Pregnant women should also practice gentle panting; this is used to help stop pushing as the baby's head is crowning (encircled by and ready to pass through the opening of the vagina).

Massage and stretching

Massage can be of great help during labor. Back massage is good for backache and also gives considerable relief if contractions are felt in the back. Leg massage is helpful against cramp (see Massage).

Yoga and stretching exercises are especially useful for pregnant women, who should practice every day for at least four months before the birth. Yoga exercises will help relaxation and strengthen the muscles used for childbirth (see Yoga).

Taking care of the appearance

If a woman looks good when she is pregnant, she will feel good too, and pregnancy actually suits a great many women.

Pregnant women should always wear comfortable clothes in flattering colors, never clothes that are too tight. Properly fitting underwear is also very important, especially a good-fitting maternity bra. Shoes should be low-heeled or flat, and women who have varicose veins should always put on support hose before getting out of bed in the morning. Keeping the hair in good condition also helps.

When a woman is pregnant, she should pay special attention to her skin during her daily routine, and use a moisturizer on her hands, neck, and face. When she takes a shower, she should massage a little baby oil into her breasts and abdomen. This will help prevent stretch marks from lingering after the birth (see Stretch Marks).

She should practice a routine of prenatal and breathing exercises for 10 minutes daily, and rest regularly to build up her energy reserves.

Prenatal classes

By the 20th week of pregnancy, the woman should enroll in a prenatal class. These classes are generally arranged by doctors and are also organized by private and charitable organizations. Again, the father of the child is welcome to attend these classes, and will be shown how best to help his partner during the course of the labor and birth.

In these classes, the growth of the fetus in its various stages will be explained. The woman and her partner will be shown exercises that aid relaxation, help prevent physical problems, and prepare the muscles that will be used in labor. Next they will be told about the whole process of birth, and may be shown a video of an actual delivery. They will also learn about labor and what to expect at each stage, including the various delivery positions, what anesthetics and analgesics (see Anesthetics; Painkillers) are available, and how to breathe correctly in order to help minimize the pain and bring about a relatively relaxed delivery.

> *See also:* **Amniocentesis; Birth; Breech birth; Exercise; Fetus; Morning sickness; Obstetrics; Preeclampsia; Pregnancy; Ultrasound; Vitamins**

Preventive medicine

"An apple a day keeps the doctor away" is obviously an oversimplification, but the principle holds true: health care and preventive medicine, both public and personal, will certainly reduce the chances of disease.

The old saying "an ounce of prevention is worth a pound of cure" has a lot of truth in it, and never more so than today, when it seems likely that the most dramatic advances in saving lives lie in preventing diseases rather than in curing them.

There are two broad categories of preventive medicine: public health or community medicine, and personal health. Public health medicine is generally concerned with such things as ensuring that water is pure, food is safe, and waste and garbage are properly disposed of.

Personal health or personal preventive medicine depends on the efforts of each individual, and is mainly concerned with making sure that a wide range of preventable disorders are avoided by having immunizations, taking safety precautions both at home and away, getting adequate sleep and exercise, and changing habits, such as smoking, that are likely to lead to disease (see Smoking). There is a strong link between public health and personal preventive medicine.

Public health

The great improvements in public health—and the associated huge leap forward in life expectancy—that took place in the first part of the last century were due not so much to advances in medical care as to the effect of considerably improved living standards (see Life Expectancy). They were also due to the control and prevention of diseases such as cholera, diphtheria, and tuberculosis by mass public health programs (see Cholera; Diphtheria; Tuberculosis).

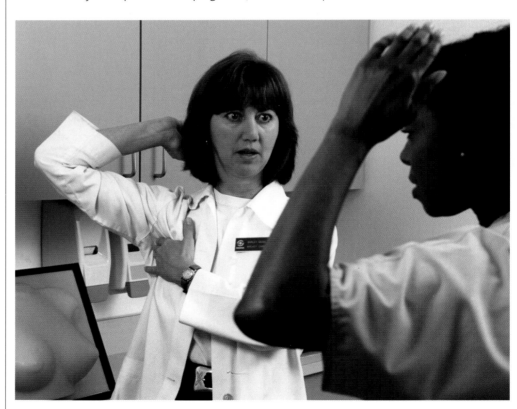

▲ *Breast cancer is one of the leading killers of women. However, a doctor can show a woman how to check her breasts for any lumps that could be malignant and thereby catch the cancer before it develops beyond the stage where it is treatable.*

Questions and Answers

I'm fed up with all this talk about health care and preventive medicine. Surely, if you give up all the things doctors want you to, life won't be worth living.

The only thing that most doctors suggest you give up altogether is smoking. Most of the other preventive measures that may be advised amount to adjustments or changes in routines, like getting additional exercise, rather than giving things up. Far from cramping their style or limiting their pleasures, most people find that adopting a simple, sensible program for taking care of the only life they have actually increases their zest for living.

Are regular medical health checkups really worthwhile?

Yes, there is growing evidence that they are. Many potentially serious conditions can be detected by examinations and tests before they give rise to any symptoms, and if treatment is given at this time the chances of either curing the condition or preventing it from developing are much higher.

What can I do during my pregnancy to help ensure that my baby is healthy?

Don't put on too much weight—eating enough for two is a myth and will spoil your figure afterward. Get enough exercise, probably more than you would normally, and get plenty of rest and sleep, particularly during the final three months. Make sure that you have your prenatal checkups and try to attend the classes. Avoid smoking altogether because it can seriously harm the baby. Alcohol should be avoided as well. However, there is no need to give up intercourse during pregnancy; not only does it not harm the baby, but it gives you and you partner some scope for inventiveness.

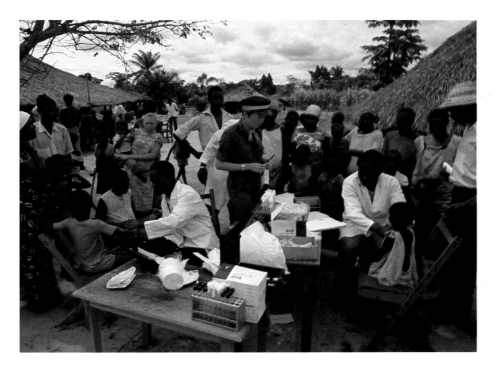

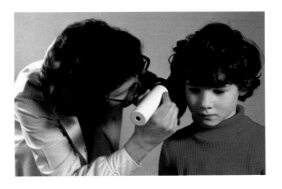

▲ *People living in some developing countries have benefited enormously from medical care and public health measures that prevent unnecessary death.*

▲ *Worldwide campaigns have made the public aware that good dental care will prevent tooth decay and gum disease.*

Of course, the continued maintenance of high standards of public health remains vital to people's safety and health. No one needs to be reminded of the vicious and devastating nature of the epidemics that do still occur from time to time when the vigilance of the public health authorities slackens (see Plague).

The second big leap forward in public health took place in the middle part of the 20th century and was based on the discovery of powerful new lifesaving drugs, particularly antibiotics. The development of radically new surgical techniques and substantial improvements in prenatal and infant welfare were also important. However, there is still room for further advances to be made in all these fields.

Personal preventive medicine

The real potential growth area in lifesaving lies in a different direction. For although the field of preventive medicine at the public level has been mined extensively, people have hardly begun to understand the possibilities in the field of personal health, let alone to exploit them.

Personal health is currently the most potent weapon people have in the crusade against unnecessary death and disability, and holds promise of saving more lives than any other area of medical advance.

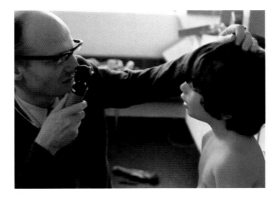

▲ *Routine eye tests are imperative to detect problems with vision which, because their onset is so gradual, are likely to be ignored.*

▼ *The ear is one of our most complex and sensitive organs, and it is prone to problems. Regular examination is very important.*

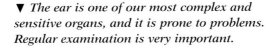

What is more, it is not a field in which humankind is waiting for some crucial new discovery or some major breakthrough in technique; it is simply a question of applying what is already known.

Early diagnosis

Early diagnosis is an area of preventive medicine that holds enormous lifesaving potential. Many people die unnecessarily, not because they have a disease for which there is no cure, but because they do not go to their doctor for investigation and treatment soon enough.

One hundred years ago most deaths occurred because no effective treatment was available for most serious illnesses, and, in these circumstances, failure to diagnose disease early made little difference to the outcome. Today, with the rapid advances in medical treatment, early diagnosis is vital in preventing unnecessary deaths, because many of the modern treatments are curative only if they are applied in the first stages of the condition. Therefore, many deaths, permanent disabilities, and cases of chronic ill health are due not to the inability of doctors to effect a cure, but to delay on the patient's part in seeking medical attention early enough to benefit fully from current techniques.

Is it good preventive medicine to stop eating fatty foods?

It is certainly good preventive medicine to take care about what you eat, but there is no reason to avoid fatty foods altogether. Many doctors believe that eating foods rich in saturated (animal) fats or in cholesterol increases the risk of developing heart and circulatory diseases, although most of the cholesterol in the blood is produced by the body itself. What is important in healthy eating is to have a nourishing diet in which the five essential ingredients—carbohydrates, fats, proteins, vitamins, and minerals—are all present in well-balanced quantities, and to remember that all foods taken in excess of what your body can utilize will turn into fat.

Does an apple a day really keep the doctor away?

Not exactly, but taking sensible care of your health certainly does. What is most likely to keep you out of the doctor's office is staying away as far as possible from smoking, underexercising, overeating, and stress. Daily fruit and vegetables certainly help.

Is it a good idea to have inoculations before going abroad?

Many parts of the world, particularly countries outside North America and Europe, do have health hazards, such as yellow fever or typhoid. It is good sense to have inoculations if you are traveling to countries where certain diseases are endemic.

If I take care of myself, will I live longer?

Life expectancy is determined by heredity, environment, and how long you have already lived. By taking precautions you will remain healthier longer, and with luck you will reach your maximum life span. The single most important thing you can do to live longer is to avoid smoking.

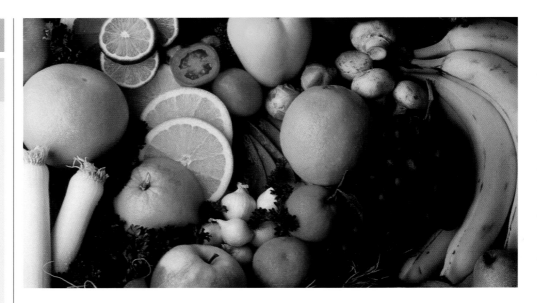

▲ *A balanced, healthy diet may not prevent illness by itself, but it can help keep the body fit and ready to fight off any problems that might occur.*

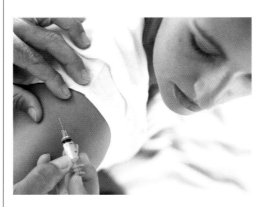

▲ *Throughout their early years and until they leave school, children are given immunizations to prevent them from catching certain diseases.*

▼ *Blood pressure problems affect many people and are a major cause of ill health. Advances in equipment now allow patients to monitor their own blood pressure.*

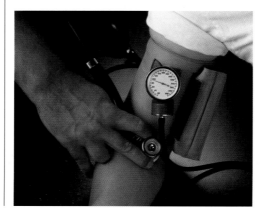

Health education

It is clear that the limiting factor in many cases of illness today lies not in what the doctor can do, but in whether the patient comes to him or her in time. A surefire method of helping to persuade people to seek medical help early is therefore likely to be even more effective in saving lives than some new medical discoveries. The prime aim of health education is to make people more aware of what they can do for themselves by increasing their knowledge of what makes them tick, and by telling them about how they themselves can affect their own health.

According to the American Heart Association's *Heart Disease and Stroke Statistics—2004 Update*, heart disease is the major cause of death in the United States; it killed 931,108 in 2001. Other major causes of death were cancer, 553,768; stroke, which accounted for more than one out of every 15 deaths; Alzheimer's disease, 53,852; and HIV, 14,175.

Of avoidable deaths, accidents accounted for 35.7 deaths per 100,000 population. Of the 101,537 deaths from accidents in 2001, 43,788 were caused by motor vehicle accidents. Motor vehicle fatality rates were 15.4 deaths per 100,000 population.

Mortality in the first year of life has dropped from 23 percent at the beginning of the 20th century to only 6.8 deaths for every 1,000 live births of all origins in 2001. Infant mortality rates ranged from 3.2 per 1,000 live births for Chinese mothers to 5.7 for white mothers to 13.3 for black mothers. Deaths among children

PREVENTIVE MEDICINE

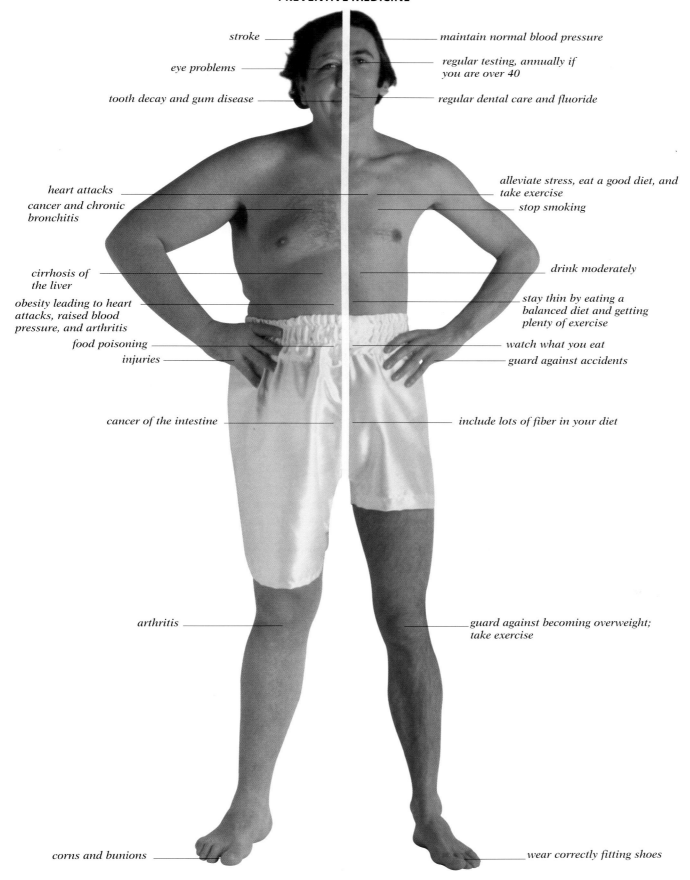

stroke ———— ———— maintain normal blood pressure

eye problems ———— ———— regular testing, annually if you are over 40

tooth decay and gum disease ———— ———— regular dental care and fluoride

heart attacks ———— ———— alleviate stress, eat a good diet, and take exercise

cancer and chronic bronchitis ———— ———— stop smoking

cirrhosis of the liver ———— ———— drink moderately

obesity leading to heart attacks, raised blood pressure, and arthritis ———— ———— stay thin by eating a balanced diet and getting plenty of exercise

food poisoning ———— ———— watch what you eat

injuries ———— ———— guard against accidents

cancer of the intestine ———— ———— include lots of fiber in your diet

arthritis ———— ———— guard against becoming overweight; take exercise

corns and bunions ———— ———— wear correctly fitting shoes

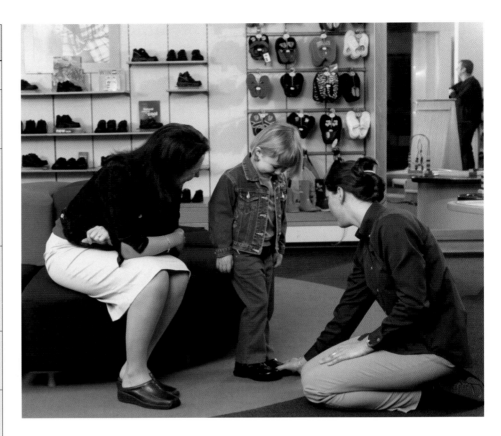

▲ *Foot problems in adults are very often the result of wearing ill-fitting shoes from childhood onward; this is why taking proper measurements is so important.*

between the ages of 1 and 14 dropped in the same period from nearly 86,000 per year to under 13,000 per year. This decrease was due mainly to the control of tuberculosis, measles, whooping cough, and diphtheria (see Measles; Whooping Cough).

Preventive medicine for all
Achievements in the control and prevention of infectious diseases tell a remarkable success story (see Infection and Infectious Diseases). The development and implementation of immunization techniques are partly responsible, as is the important part played by measures designed to prevent the organisms that cause disease from ever reaching the body, particularly the public health measures that are implemented to ensure the safety of food and water, and the efficient disposal of sewage. However, outbreaks of preventable diseases—especially gastrointestinal infections—will still occur unless adequate personal and domestic hygiene is maintained (see Food Poisoning).

Checkups
Many people wonder whether regular medical checkups are a worthwhile preventive measure. It is true that people can drop dead on their way home from a health checkup at which nothing was found wrong with them, because some serious conditions cannot be detected by any form of screening. It is also true that not all doctors agree about the validity of checkups; some feel that abnormalities found, for example, in blood tests do not necessarily indicate that the person will develop a disease if nothing is done about them.

On the other hand, there is no doubt that regular checkups do pick up unsuspected conditions that may require treatment, and

conceivably save lives. This fact alone makes regular checkups well worth doing. The areas in which regular checks are most important are the eyes, ears, teeth, weight, heart and circulation, lungs, urine, and blood, plus breasts and a gynecological examination for women (see Breasts; Internal Examination). The ideal person to carry out a health check is the family doctor, since he or she is probably the only person who knows enough about the patient to be able to put the findings into the right perspective.

Health checks are not always covered by health insurance plans. Nevertheless, many doctors are prepared to do them, much as they will carry out medical examinations for either insurance or employment purposes, and for a similar fee.

Health checks are carried out routinely on children throughout their school years, and the suggested frequency in adult life, when they are done on a voluntary basis, is every five years until the age of 45, and every one or two years after that.

Maintaining health
An apple a day doesn't necessarily keep the doctor away, but the golden rule in personal preventive medicine is for people to take the best possible care of their health, which should include eating a well-balanced diet with plenty of fruit and vegetables—this is the thread that should run throughout life (see Diet).

See also: Accident prevention; Antibiotics; Dental care; Diagnosis; Exercise; Health care system; Health education; Hygiene; Immunization; Prenatal care; Public health

Prickly heat

If a person goes to a tropical climate and reacts to the heat by sweating profusely, he or she may develop prickly heat—a rash characterized by small red spots and intense itching that is caused by blockage of the sweat ducts.

Questions and Answers

I'm planning a trip to the tropics, where I previously got prickly heat. How can I avoid it this time?

Let your body acclimatize slowly to the hot, humid climate. If possible, stay in air-conditioned rooms for the first few days, then go out only for an hour or so for the next few days. This should build up your tolerance gradually until you can go out in the heat with minimal sweating. Wear loose cotton clothes. Take vitamin C daily; it may help the skin resist the heat.

My daughter gets rashes easily. Is this prickly heat?

Probably not. Babies often get rashes when they have a fever. These are usually not prickly heat, but the treatment is the same; keep your baby cool and dress her in loose clothes. In the first weeks of life, babies often develop rashes on the face and trunk that look like prickly heat; make sure you avoid high temperatures in the nursery.

Last summer I got prickly spots on my arms after sunbathing. Why?

Many sun lotions block the sweat pores so that subsequent sweating goes into the skin, causing a type of prickly heat. Try to accustom your skin slowly to the sun, rather than going out on the first day and relying on the protection of suntan oil. It is also possible to develop an allergy rash to sun lotions, but this is an itchy red rash rather than the tiny pricking spots of prickly heat.

I developed prickly heat after spending a month in the tropics. Why the delay?

In prickly heat, sweat blocks the sweat ducts instead of coming to the surface and evaporating. It can take a month of excessive washing, friction from clothes, and further sweating to develop prickly heat.

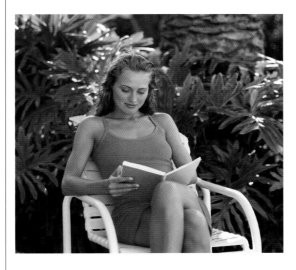

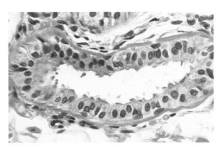

◄▲ *Prickly heat results when the sweat gland ducts (above) become blocked with sweat. Keeping cool, by acclimatizing slowly and wearing loose cotton clothes (left), is the most effective form of prevention.*

Prickly heat is an itchy skin rash that occurs on exposure to extreme heat and humidity. Although virtually unknown in people with dark complexions, prickly heat affects 30 percent of Caucasians when they visit tropical climates. Children are particularly prone to this irritating condition.

Causes
Prickly heat is due to the obstruction of the sweat gland ducts in the skin. Sweat is forced into the tissues immediately under the skin, and, since sweat is an irritant, it sets up a reaction that causes the rash. A vicious circle is created: the sweat damages the skin; this damage then gives rise to prickly heat, which further damages the skin, exacerbating the condition.

Symptoms and dangers
The worst-affected areas are those where skin damage from friction and sweat are most likely. These include the neck, armpits, groin, waistband, backs of knees, and fronts of the elbows. Large numbers of minute red spots arise, accompanied by a characteristic pricking sensation. When the skin cools, the symptoms subside, but if nothing is done to relieve the continuing skin damage from the friction and the sweating, recurrent episodes that last several days will occur.

In some cases the damaged skin may become infected, producing spreading redness, pain, and even pus. When this occurs, antibiotic treatment may be necessary (see Antibiotics).

Treatment and outlook
The cure for prickly heat is to stop the sweating. This usually means staying in air-conditioned rooms. Loose clothes should be worn to prevent friction; cotton is preferable to synthetics, which cause sweating. Soap and other skin irritants should be avoided, since these increase itching; and frequent showers will only make the problem worse. Although there are numerous other treatments, none will be effective unless the sweating is reduced. In the meantime, calamine lotion will help relieve the prickling.

Eventually, the body will acclimatize to the heat and the attacks will lessen. However, someone who has suffered from prickly heat before will usually get it again on returning to tropical climates.

See also: Heat and heat disorders; Itches; Perspiration; Rashes

Prolapse

Questions and Answers

When my gynecologist examined me, she said I had a small prolapse of the uterus. I have not noticed any problems but am worried that I may eventually need surgery.

Many women, especially in their later years, have some degree of prolapse, but there is no need to treat it unless it causes problems.

My husband and I are in our fifties and still enjoy sex together. I am about to have an operation for a prolapse. Will this interfere with our lovemaking?

Discuss this beforehand with the surgeon. Pieces of loose tissue are usually removed from the vagina as part of the surgery, making the vagina narrower. The vagina is left wide enough, however, to allow you to continue to enjoy sex.

My nine-year-old nephew is suffering from a prolapsed rectum. Will he need surgery?

Rectal prolapse in children is not usually serious and can often be pushed back or reduced without too much discomfort.

My elderly mother had a prolapse of her uterus that has been corrected with a ring pessary. She is supposed to go to the hospital every six months to have a new pessary, but finds it difficult to get there. Would it matter if she did not have the pessary changed, since she has no trouble with it?

Most women with ring pessaries dislike having them changed because they find the experience uncomfortable and embarrassing. These pessaries can cause an unpleasant vaginal discharge or vaginal ulcers that bleed. This is why a clean one needs to be fitted every six months. One bonus is that the doctor may find that your mother no longer needs a pessary.

Prolapse means literally "to slip downward" and can be applied to any organ in the body that has been displaced from its normal position because of weakness in the supporting tissues.

The fibrous and muscular sling that lies across the bones forming the pelvic girdle is called the pelvic floor. This has to support the weight of all the contents of the abdominal cavity, such as the gut and the bladder, and, in women, the uterus as well. Occasionally, if the support system is weakened, the uterus may slide down into the vagina. This is called a uterine prolapse.

The vaginal wall is surrounded by many important structures that can also lose their support and bulge into the vagina. When the intestine bulges into the vagina, it is called an enterocele or rectocele, depending on which part of the intestine is involved. When the bladder prolapses into the vagina the condition is called a cystocele, and when the urethra loses its supports it is described as a urethrocele (see Bladder and Bladder Problems; Urethra). All these conditions are forms of prolapse, and more than one of them will usually exist in the same woman.

Causes

Anything that exerts too much weight or pressure on the pelvic floor, or weakens it, will make a woman more likely to develop a prolapse: for example, coughing, heavy lifting, or regular straining on defecation. Frequent pregnancies, especially if the babies are large or if labor is prolonged, will weaken the mother's pelvic floor, as will obesity in a woman (see Obesity).

The supporting tissues seem to need a hormone called estrogen to retain their strength (see Estrogen; Hormones). This is released mainly from a woman's ovaries. After menopause, the ovaries no longer secrete large amounts of estrogen (see Menopause; Ovaries). The pelvic floor becomes weaker and, as a result, the woman is in greater danger of developing a prolapse at this time.

Symptoms of uterine prolapse

The symptoms a prolapse produces depend on its severity and whether or not the bladder or intestine is involved. Many women have no symptoms; some simply experience a downward

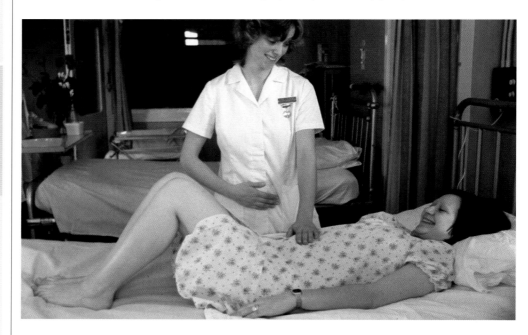

▲ *Teaching a new mother exercises to strengthen her pelvic floor is an important part of postnatal care, since it can prevent prolapse of the uterus in later life.*

pressure in the vagina. Others feel a lump (the uterus) in the vagina or complain of feeling something coming down. In a few cases, the entire uterus protrudes from the vagina. Obviously, this makes walking and sitting very uncomfortable, but it is very uncommon. If the intestine is involved in the prolapse, the woman may find it difficult to defecate without pushing the uterus back into the vagina. The same is true if the bladder is part of the prolapse. However, a much more common problem is that the woman finds that she leaks urine if she runs, laughs, or coughs. This is called stress incontinence.

A prolapse of the uterus does not cause any vaginal bleeding or pain, but occasionally women may notice a dull backache at the end of the day, which is relieved by lying down.

Prolapses are becoming less common, partly because women have better nutrition and tend to have smaller families, but largely owing to better prenatal preparation (see Prenatal Care).

Prevention of uterine prolapse

It is important to try to prevent prolapses. The muscles of the pelvic floor can be strengthened by Kegel exercises; women both at prenatal classes and in the maternity suite are taught these exercises. It is not always easy for a mother of a young baby to find the time to perform the exercises, but it is important for her future that she try to spare a few minutes daily. Weight loss often helps reduce the risk of prolapse. A high-fiber diet will make bowel movements easier. Not partaking in activities that stress pelvic support muscles can also help.

Treatment

If a woman's prolapse is very small but she is overweight, it can sometimes be corrected if she loses weight and is prescribed a course of exercise treatment by a physical therapist. Elderly or unfit women who wish to avoid surgery for more severe forms of prolapse can be treated by placing a plastic or rubber ring (a ring pessary) in the vagina to hold the uterus in place. Fit women with severe symptoms are usually advised to have surgery. There are several types of surgery, but they are almost all performed on or through the vagina so that the woman has no visible scar (see Surgery).

Other forms of prolapse

Although it is customary to think of a prolapse as something that affects only the uterus in women, there are other structures in the body that can prolapse or slip downward.

RECTAL PROLAPSE

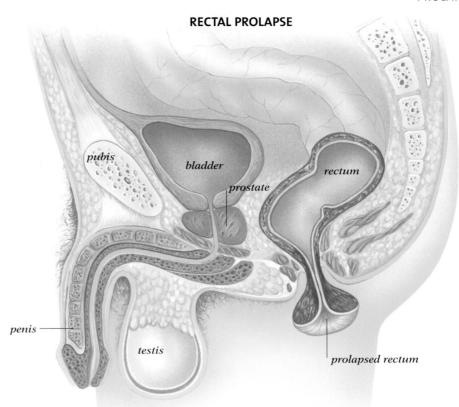

▲ *In rectal prolapse the rectum protrudes from the anus. While men and women may need an operation, in children the prolapse can be pushed back without much discomfort.*

▼ *A prolapse of the bladder and urethra into the vagina often leads to urine leakage, which occurs when a woman runs, laughs, or coughs (this is called stress incontinence).*

PROLAPSE OF THE BLADDER AND URETHRA

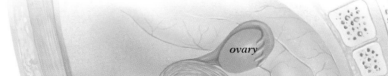

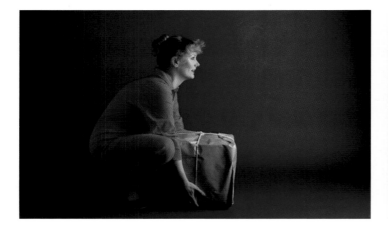
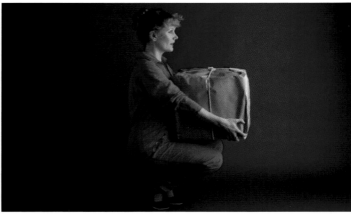
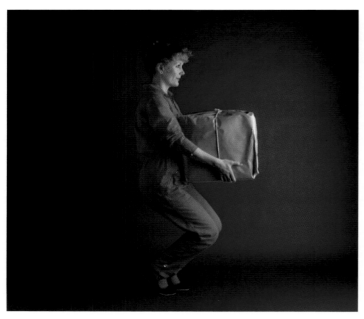
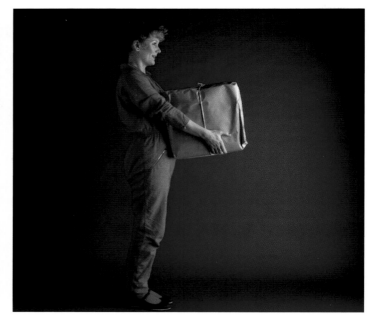

▲ *To avoid straining the pelvic floor, it is important to lift heavy objects correctly. Bend at the knees and, keeping your back straight, use your arm muscles to lift the object. Then use your leg muscles to help you straighten up again.*

One of the most dramatic but rare forms is a prolapsed cord. In the process of birth a baby's umbilical cord comes out of the birth canal first, before the baby, and may be compressed against the bones of the mother's pelvis, thus interfering with the supply of blood to the baby. Special measures are needed to deal with this and to ensure that the baby survives unharmed (see Cesarean Birth).

Doctors also talk about a prolapsed intervertebral disk. Normally this is called a "slipped disk"; the term means that one of the spongy middle sections of the tough disks that lie between the vertebrae has broken through the fibrous ring that surrounds it, and is pressing on a nerve leaving the spinal cord.

After uterine prolapse, the most common sort of prolapse is that of the rectum. The rectum is pushed down through the anal orifice. Since the rectum is a tube that is actually tethered to the anus, it can be pushed down through it like a sock being turned inside out. This happens more often in women than in men, but it also happens in children. The condition is not usually serious in children, and the prolapse can nearly always be reduced (pushed back) without too much discomfort, and usually without the need for surgery. In adults, however, there is often a need to operate and the prolapse cannot be reduced so easily. For a severe prolapse, it is usually necessary to open the abdomen and repair the damage from the inside. It is unclear why rectal prolapse occurs. In children, constipation and excessive straining to defecate may be a cause (see Constipation). In adults, the condition is usually found in elderly women, although it also occurs in men at any age. A laxity of the muscles of the floor of the pelvis may be a part of the cause, although the rectum does not seem more likely to prolapse if women have had a lot of children.

Outlook

It is usually possible to cure a prolapse of the uterus completely. In a small percentage of women, however, the symptoms may recur years later, so it is important for a woman who has been successfully treated once to avoid putting too much strain on her pelvic floor in the future.

See also: Anus; Back and backache; Gynecology; Incontinence; Pelvis; Physical therapy; Rectum; Slipped disk; Uterus; Vagina

Prostaglandins

Questions and Answers

My son has some sort of allergy to food which we think is caused by milk. Could prostaglandins give rise to his symptoms?

It is possible. Prostaglandins belong to a group of transmitting substances, some of which are involved in allergies. Recent research has shown that certain allergic reactions to food can be blocked by aspirin; this suggests that prostaglandins are involved in some cases.

Is it true that prostaglandins can cause heart attacks?

One type of prostaglandin is vital for making blood-clotting cells, or platelets, stick together to form a clot. This process may be a factor in forming blockages in the coronary arteries that lead to heart attacks. However, there is another prostaglandin that acts to reduce clotting. Prostaglandin-blocking drugs, such as aspirin, have real value in helping to prevent heart attacks by reducing the risk of thrombosis, but the major cause of heart attacks is the arterial disease atherosclerosis, which affects the coronary arteries and forms plaque sites on which blood is likely to clot.

Could my body work without prostaglandins?

Almost certainly not. They are essential in many ways, especially in dealing with injury and infection, and they may have other, as yet unknown, roles.

I have arthritis. Should I take prostaglandin-blocking drugs?

You may already be taking them. Most common painkillers have some prostaglandin-blocking activities. There are many new drugs available, but the older ones are still as effective.

Prostaglandins are chemical substances that are similar to hormones; they act as messengers in the body and are responsible for controlling many important physical functions.

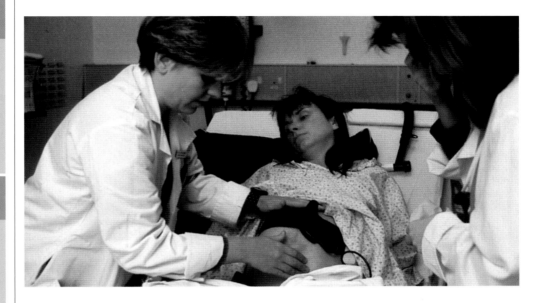

▲ *Prostaglandins E2 and F2 can stimulate muscle contractions during labor. They may be given in the form of pessaries to help speed up or induce labor.*

When prostaglandins arrive at a cell or tissue that is primed to respond to them, they trigger an important reaction. Unlike hormones, they are not produced just in specialized glands but may be produced in different tissues. Their effect is on cells and tissues nearby.

Discovery of prostaglandins

Prostaglandins were first found in the prostate gland, hence the name. Because they have a short lifetime (a few seconds between production and effect), they are difficult to study. They may not even enter the bloodstream, and so it is very difficult to measure the amounts of active prostaglandin that may be present. Most of the prostaglandins that have been found so far were discovered because they can produce a measurable effect on tissue samples in a laboratory.

How prostaglandins work

Many different body tissues respond to prostaglandins. They are central to the female reproductive system, and may help regulate menstrual bleeding. Menstrual pain may result from an imbalance in prostaglandins. Prostaglandins are relevant to men; a deficiency in seminal fluid is thought to reduce male fertility. Prostaglandins are associated with common aches and pains, as well as severe inflammation of arthritis. Aspirin, an effective painkiller, blocks prostaglandin production, and a range of more powerful drugs use the same principle. Prostaglandins produced by blood platelets are also closely involved with blood clotting and blood thinning.

There are many different prostaglandins; and each has a different effect, so creating drugs to manipulate them is a delicate process. For example, aspirin will reduce heart and circulatory problems by preventing blood clots, but it will block the production of prostaglandins that protect the stomach lining, and it may cause ulcers and stomach upsets. New drugs are being developed to block specific prostaglandins, and allow others to function normally.

See also: Arthritis; Hormones; Painkillers

Prostate gland

Questions and Answers

What is the function of the prostate gland, and can it be removed safely?

It produces a special fluid that makes up part of the seminal fluid and allows the sperm to remain active, probably increasing the chances of fertilization. The prostate gland can be removed successfully without any adverse effect on health, although fertility and sexual performance may be affected. Because this operation is usually performed on elderly men, they may not care about infertility.

My father has been told he has prostate cancer, but his physicians are not going to operate. Does this mean that it has spread too far?

A high proportion of prostate cancers in older men are confined to the gland, progress very slowly, and do no harm. A "watchful waiting" policy is often adopted by urologists and is usually justified.

Do the hormones used to treat prostate cancer have side effects?

Yes, in some patients, but these are rarely serious enough to stop the treatment. They include increased retention of fluid in the tissues, enlargement of breast tissue, and loss of body hair and libido.

My husband is developing difficulty in urinating. He has to stand for ages before the urine starts to flow, and he is getting up several times a night. Does he need an operation on his prostate gland?

Possibly. There are other causes of the same symptoms, but he should see a specialist to have some tests carried out, including a blood test, a special X ray, and a urine flow test. These tests reveal whether or not the prostate gland is the cause of the trouble. If it is, surgery would be recommended.

The main function of the prostate gland is to aid male fertility. It is common for this gland to remain relatively trouble-free until late in life, and if problems do occur, they can usually be treated successfully.

The prostate gland is a walnut-shaped structure found only in males. It is situated at the base of the bladder and surrounds the urethra, the tube through which urine and seminal fluid pass out of the body. This gland produces the fluid that mixes with semen to make up part of the seminal fluid. Although the full function of the prostatic fluid is unknown, one of its roles is to help keep the sperm active so that fertilization can occur more easily.

Owing to its position in the body, problems associated with this gland can often affect the functioning of the bladder, though this condition is more common among elderly men.

Prostate problems

There are various things that can go wrong with the prostate gland during a man's lifetime. The gland can become inflamed as a result of bacterial infection (see Bacteria). This condition, known as acute prostatitis, causes flulike symptoms and pain in the lower abdomen, groin, and perineum (tissue between the anus and external genitalia). More rarely, there may be a discharge from the

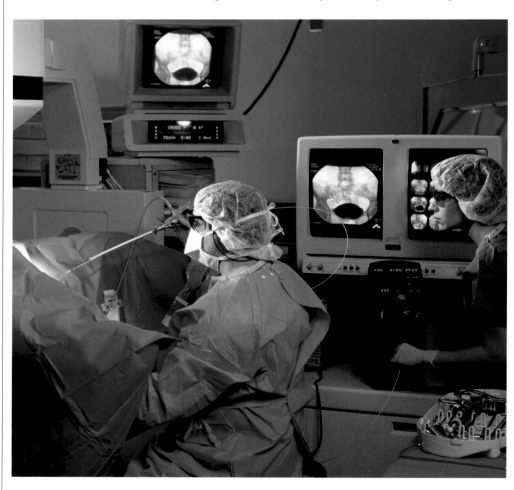

▲ *A surgeon performs minimally invasive interstitial (indigo) laser surgery on a patient with an enlarged prostate. The operation takes 30–60 minutes and uses a cystoscope to emit heat through a fiber-optic probe, thereby destroying the excess prostate tissue.*

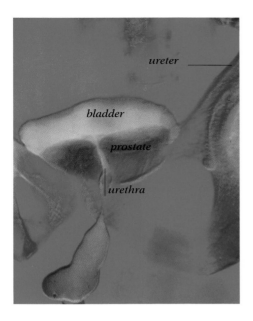

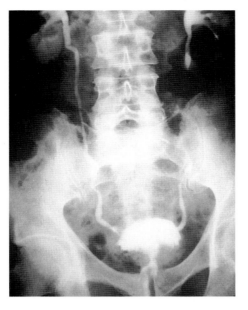

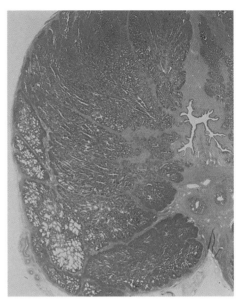

▲ *The state of the prostate gland, whether it is enlarged or not, can be determined by means of special X-ray techniques. A normal-size gland can be seen in the cystogram (above left) and an enlarged gland in the pyelogram (above right).*

▲ *As seen in this micrograph, the prostate is made up of glandular tissue and smooth muscle fibers.*

penis. Occasionally, this infection can lead to an abscess in the gland (see Abscess), or to chronic prostatitis if there is a persistent low-grade infection.

As a result of chronic prostatitis, the gland may become calcified and gravel-like stones may be formed. Prostatitis is treated with antibiotics, although recurrent problems are common (see Antibiotics). Surgery may be required to treat the abscess. Another problem that can affect the prostate gland is the development of a tumor. The treatment of this condition varies, depending on whether the tumor is benign or malignant (see Tumors).

Signs of a benign enlargement

The most common disorder of the prostate gland is a benign increase in the size of the gland. This noncancerous condition affects many elderly men, although young men can suffer from it too.

Benign enlargement of the prostate gland (hyperplasia) is so common that many doctors believe that every man over the age of about 50 years has some degree of hyperplasia; it just has to be accepted as part of the aging process (see Aging).

Because the prostate gland surrounds the urethra, and because it is so close to the base of the bladder, enlargement of the gland can seriously impair the normal mechanism of urination. A man with an enlarged prostate may notice the following symptoms: increased frequency of urination during the day; getting up at night to urinate; the development of a poor urinary stream; a tendency to stop and start, with the sensation that there is more to come; having to wait several seconds before urine starts to flow; dribbling of urine after the stream; and sometimes a sudden urge to urinate.

All these symptoms are due to distortion of the normal anatomy at the base of the bladder. The enlargement of the gland squeezes the urethra, causing it to become narrow. Sometimes the central

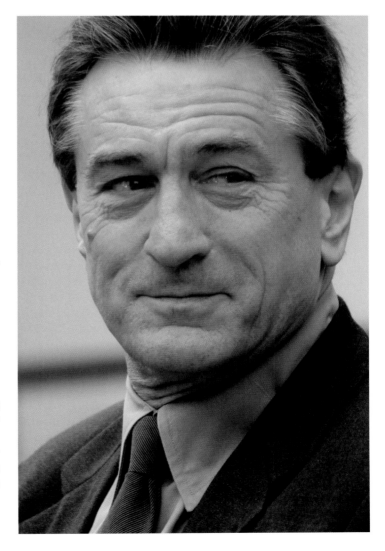

▶ *The actor Robert De Niro was diagnosed with prostate cancer during a routine medical test in October 2003.*

Questions and Answers

Why does the prostate gland become enlarged in older men?

No one really knows the answer to this. Finding an enlarged prostate gland is so common that it is difficult to equate it with factors earlier in life, such as sexual activity.

Is removal of the prostate gland using an open operation likely to be more permanent in its effect than removal with an instrument through the penis?

It can be, but doesn't have to be. Removal of the gland can be complete when done by the closed method, that is, by a transurethral resection (TURP), where a fine tube complete with a viewing piece and a cautery device is introduced into the penis and the prostate is actually chipped away. However, using the TURP method, some surgeons might only remove part of the gland in a very old person, just so that he can urinate easily.

Can anything be done for the pain in the bones that my father suffers as a result of his prostatic cancer spreading?

Yes. If hormone treatment has been tried and has not been successful, radiotherapy of the painful area is often extremely effective in relieving the pain of secondary tumors in the bones. Some experts also recommend removal of the testes, since this will decrease levels of testosterone and may cause the tumor to shrink.

I am due to have a prostatectomy soon. Is there a chance that I will be incontinent after I have my prostate gland removed?

There is a very small chance of this in the first few months after the operation because the muscles of the bladder that prevent leakage may be damaged during the operation, but it usually gets better in time and the incontinence ceases.

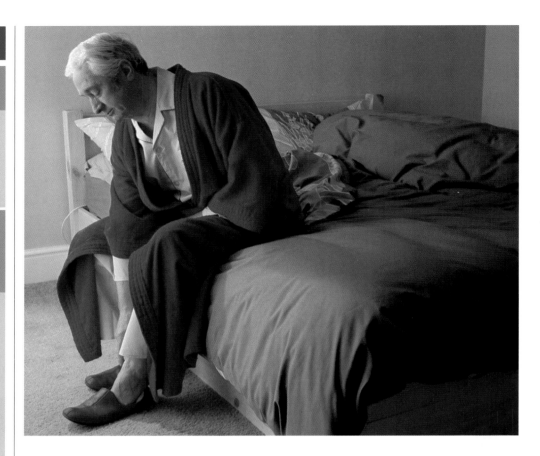

▲ *A prostatectomy relieves one of the most awkward and exhausting symptoms of an enlarged prostate gland—that is, frequent nighttime urination.*

part of the gland becomes elongated and extends up into the bladder, where it can then block the entrance to the urethra and thereby inhibit the exit of urine.

If a man continues to have these symptoms without seeking medical help, there can be a sudden and complete inability to urinate (acute retention), which is extremely painful and requires immediate treatment. A catheter (tube) has to be passed into the bladder to drain off the excess urine.

The obstruction to outflow makes it impossible to empty the bladder, so filling up to the point of discomfort occurs much more rapidly than normal. Therefore, frequent visits to the toilet, night and day, are necessary. Eventually, he urinates in a dribble, and may even find that he is continually wetting his underwear and his bed (see Incontinence).

In the end, there is so much back pressure on the kidneys that they start failing, and waste products build up in the bloodstream, with extremely serious consequences, such as high blood pressure and anemia. This situation is called chronic retention of urine with renal failure (see Kidneys and Kidney Diseases).

Treatment

When a patient goes to his doctor complaining of difficulty in urinating or, perhaps, passing small quantities frequently, he will be sent for a series of special tests, including an X ray of the kidneys and bladder, and blood tests. Special equipment may also be used to measure his urine flow.

If the tests show that the prostate gland is enlarged, surgery would be recommended, because leaving the gland to enlarge further would complicate treatment later on. An operation would also be recommended for a patient who develops acute retention of urine, since urination is possible only with the aid of a catheter. Also, a permanent bladder catheter can be a social problem—as well as a medical one, because of the increased risk of infection in the urine.

If the prostate gland is causing symptoms because it is enlarged, there are no drugs that can permanently reduce the size of the gland. Some drugs may help the symptoms to a certain extent, but they probably help only to postpone inevitable surgery.

Prostate surgery

The prostate gland is situated in an extremely inaccessible part of the body, and, because of this, surgery to remove it can be difficult. Also, because it is near the opening of the bladder, the delicate muscles that prevent urine from leaking in between the acts of urination can be damaged if great care is not taken.

There are two types of surgery: the transurethral resection of prostate (TURP), also known as the closed method; and the retropubic prostatectomy, or open method.

The closed method, or TURP, is performed using a fine telescopelike instrument called a cystoscope, which is passed up the penis into the bladder. This instrument has a viewing piece and a special cautery (searing) device that has a wire loop on the end. Using this method, the prostate gland is chipped away from inside the urethra, with little pieces of tissue being cut away each time the wire loop, which is attached to an electric current, moves through the tissue.

The great advantage of the TURP method is that the patient is spared a surgical incision and there is less discomfort or pain after the surgery. A tube is left in the bladder, which is usually taken out after two or three days. Patients make a much quicker recovery from TURP because it is less traumatic to the body than the open method.

The open method is used for very large glands and also when surgery on the bladder has to be done at the same time. It is also often used to treat cancer of the prostate. The operation consists of making a cut across the lower abdomen and approaching the gland through the space between the back of the pubic bone and the bladder.

The capsule of the prostate gland is opened and the gland is scooped out from inside the capsule. Fluid is then passed via a tube into the bladder to prevent the formation of blood clots. This tube is usually left in the bladder for about five days after the operation and then removed if there is no residual bleeding. A patient having this operation is usually in the hospital for seven to 10 days.

After a prostatectomy, the urinary stream is noticeably better, but there will be side effects. Because of the anatomy of the prostate gland, patients who have had either type of prostatectomy will find that they are unable to ejaculate semen normally. In this condition, known as retrograde ejaculation, the semen goes back into the bladder instead of traveling down and out the penis, in effect making the man infertile. This is because the muscle at the base of the bladder has to be cut when the prostate gland is removed. This muscle usually contracts during orgasm, preventing semen from going up into the bladder.

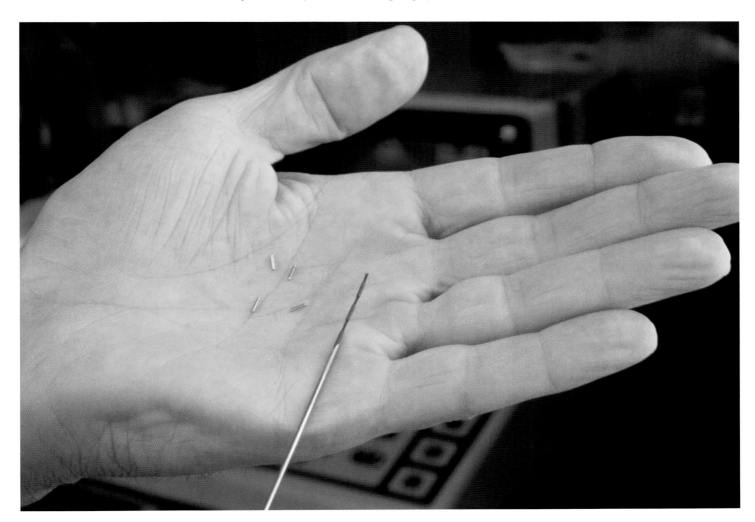

▲ *In one of the more recent treatments for early-stage prostate cancer, called ultrasound-guided prostate seed brachytherapy, radioactive seeds resembling silver rice pellets are implanted into the prostate through the skin between the scrotum and the rectum by ultrasound-guided needles. This procedure, usually given under spinal or general anesthesia, takes 45 to 90 minutes.*

▶ *The condition of the prostate gland can be diagnosed by a rectal examination. If it is enlarged, a transurethral resection (closed surgery) or a retropubic prostatectomy (open surgery) will be recommended.*

Since this surgery is usually performed on elderly men, they may not care about infertility (and sexual performance need not be affected), but a younger man suffering from an enlarged prostate may be worried by the prospect of retrograde ejaculation if he wants to have children (see Infertility). Sometimes the surgeon will be able to postpone treatment until the man has fathered a child, but this is not always possible if the symptoms are very severe. However, it is sometimes possible for the man's partner to be artificially inseminated if desired (see Artificial Methods of Conception).

Cancer of the prostate

Cancer of the prostate is one of the most common cancers to occur in males. In fact, it has been found in routine postmortem examinations that nearly all elderly men have a tiny mass of cancer in the prostate gland. Most of these men would not have known that they had anything wrong. However, when a malignant tumor does manifest itself during a man's life, it does so in a number of ways (see Malignancy). First, it may be found on a routine examination by a doctor who notices a lump in the gland (the gland can be felt through the anterior wall of the rectum). Second, the patient may have difficulty passing urine because the tumor is so close to the urethra. Third, the patient may have no urinary symptoms, but develops symptoms from the spread of the tumor outside the gland. One of the most common sites for the secondary spread of the tumor is in the bones. The spread results when tiny clumps of cells break off the main tumor and circulate in the bloodstream.

Treatment and outlook

The treatment of cancer of the prostate depends on many factors, but one of the most important is the spreading of the tumor. Therefore, a patient who is suspected of having a malignant tumor of the prostate will have several tests, including X rays and radioactive scans of the bones, to determine the exact extent of the spread (see Scans; X Rays). If the tumor has been found by accident, and consists of a small nodule confined to the gland itself, most surgeons would treat this by removing the prostate.

If the tests show that the tumor has spread outside the prostate gland, then treatment in the form of hormone drugs will be given (see Hormones). Most cancers of the prostate have been found to be dependent on male hormones for their growth; so by counteracting their effect with estrogen, a female hormone, the cancer can be kept at bay (see Estrogen). The drug is given in very small doses and often has dramatic effects on the primary and secondary tumors. Bones

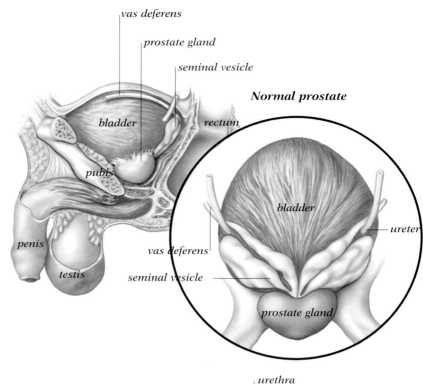

Normal prostate

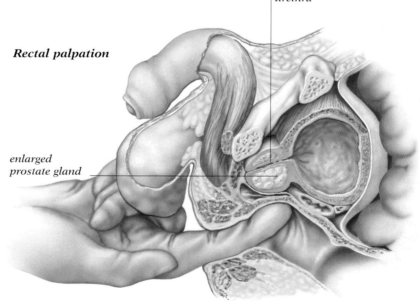

Rectal palpation

that have been riddled with secondary tumors become normal again, and the swelling in the gland becomes smaller.

The female hormone drug does have side effects, however, which some patients may find worrying. It can decrease libido, promote the loss of hair, and increase the growth of breast tissue (see Libido). It can also cause the body tissues to retain more fluid than usual, leading to swelling of the ankles (see Edema), and sometimes to heart failure.

A more recent treatment, now widely used, is the drug bicalutamide (Casodex). This drug blocks the male hormone receptors on the prostate cells and significantly reduces the tendency for the cancer to grow. It has largely replaced estrogen and

TREATMENT OF PROSTATE PROBLEMS

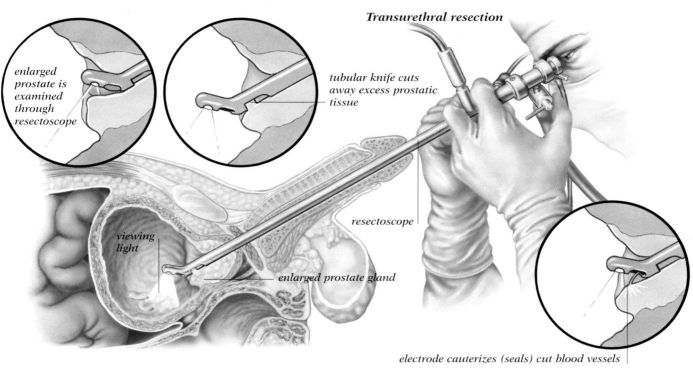

Transurethral resection

enlarged prostate is examined through resectoscope

tubular knife cuts away excess prostatic tissue

resectoscope

viewing light

enlarged prostate gland

electrode cauterizes (seals) cut blood vessels

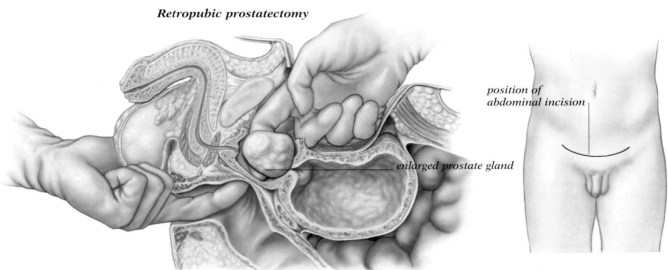

Retropubic prostatectomy

position of abdominal incision

enlarged prostate gland

has reduced the necessity to remove the testes—the source of the male hormones (see Testes). Casodex is, however, likely to cause breast enlargement (gynecomastia), tiredness, loss of libido, and other side effects.

A recent treatment for prostate cancer that is in the early stage is seed brachytherapy, in which radioactive seeds are implanted in the prostate by needles that are guided by ultrasound.

No treatment may be recommended if the patient is elderly, if he has a limited life expectancy, and if the cancer is small and confined to the prostate gland. This is because many such patients will die from other unrelated causes without experiencing any symptoms as a result of their cancer, and surgery is an unnecessary ordeal.

There are a small number of patients whose tumors do not respond to drug treatment. Luckily, they are a very small proportion of patients with cancer of the prostate. The outlook for many patients with prostatic cancer is good. Some men live an active life for years, taking a small dose of the hormone drug daily.

See also: **Bladder and bladder problems; Cancer; Erection and ejaculation; Genitals; Penis and disorders; Semen; Sperm; Testosterone; Urethra; Urinary tract and disorders**

Prostheses

Thanks to the development of new technology and to improved surgical techniques, many parts of the body—from arms to heart valves—can now be replaced. These replacement devices are called prostheses.

Questions and Answers

I have had severe pain in my right hip for several years now and my doctor says that it is due to arthritis. He thinks I should have an artificial hip joint fitted, but I am worried because it sounds like major surgery. What do you advise?

If you are troubled with severe pain, a hip replacement would give you dramatic relief. It is a big but routine operation, and the overall results are very good. Your life could be completely transformed.

What kind of deafness can be treated by the insertion of metal or plastic bones into the middle ear?

This treatment is used for deafness caused by the seizing up of a chain of tiny bones in the middle ear, a condition called otosclerosis. Sometimes injuries to the ear can be helped by a similar operation. Deafness caused by damage or disease of the nerve that conveys the impulses from the ear to the brain would not be helped at all.

How do the joints of an artificial leg work?

In the leg, the joints are fairly basic. The knee joint in an above-the-knee prosthesis can be bent and straightened. To prevent the leg collapsing when walking, there is a spring catch that engages when the leg is straight. This catch can be released when the patient wants to bend his or her knee. The ankle joint is usually fixed.

Can a new hip joint be put in if the artificial one wears out?

Yes, although the operation is often more difficult because of all the scar tissue present from the previous surgery. The artificial joints do not usually wear out, but they can loosen their attachments to the surrounding bone, and this makes movements painful again.

When a part of the body is replaced by an artificial device, that device is usually called a prosthesis (from the Greek word *prostithenai*, meaning "to put something in place of"). There are many parts of the body, both internal and external, that can be replaced, and the prostheses available today range from false teeth to artificial joints, limbs, bones, heart valves, breasts, and parts of the male genitalia (see Genitals). External replacements, such as artificial limbs, have been used for hundreds of years and have become more and more refined. However, internal prostheses, or implants, have been used only recently, mainly because in the past suitable materials were not available and surgical techniques were not sufficiently developed. With the advances in technology and the development of special plastics, silastics, and highly refined metals, these problems have, to a great extent, been overcome, and internal implants have been produced for ears, breasts, heart valves, joints, larynx, urinary sphincter, and eyes.

Artificial limbs

Artificial limbs are used to replace limbs that have had to be removed because of injury, tumor, infection, or poor blood supply (see Gangrene), and also in cases where a person has been born with a short or absent limb. There are two main problems associated with artificial limbs: how to fix the limb onto the patient, and how to control the movement of the limb.

Legs

In the case of prostheses of the lower limb, there have been many devices used to hold the limb in place. The level at which the leg has been amputated is, of course, very important. The longer

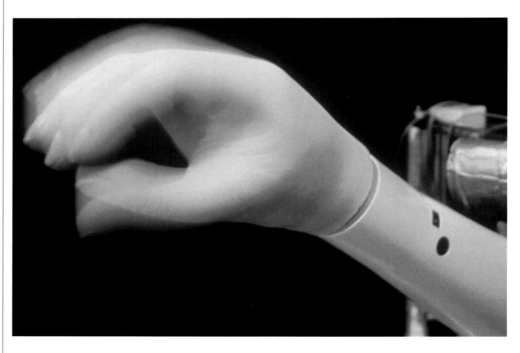

▲ *A myoelectric prosthetic arm is driven by a battery-powered electrode attached to the skin that is triggered and controlled by the user's muscle contractions (*myo *is the Greek word for "muscle"). Fitted with a hand and rotating wrist, it gives the user precise control of the limb and enables him or her to utilize skills and enjoy an active life.*

HOW A BODY-POWERED ARTIFICIAL LIMB WORKS

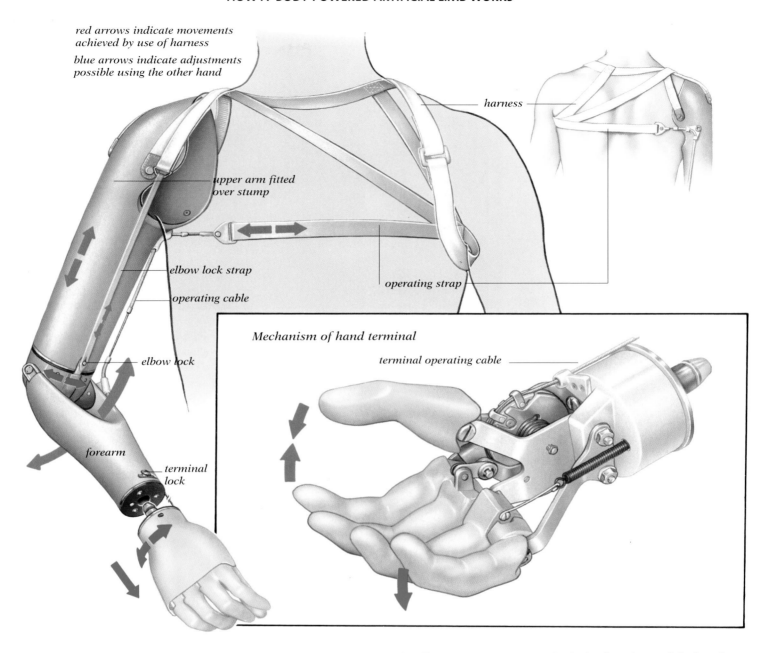

*red arrows indicate movements
achieved by use of harness*

*blue arrows indicate adjustments
possible using the other hand*

harness

upper arm fitted
over stump

elbow lock strap

operating cable

operating strap

Mechanism of hand terminal

terminal operating cable

elbow lock

forearm

terminal
lock

▲ *The prosthetic limb shown above has been designed for an above-the-elbow amputation, in which the functions of the hand, wrist, and elbow have been lost, but controlled movement of the shoulder and arm stump has been retained. Essentially, the amputee is trained to make movements of the stump, shoulder, shoulder blades, and back. By means of a series of straps and cables, these movements enable the amputee to lock and unlock the elbow unit, to move the forearm up and down, and to operate the hand or other terminal attachment. For greater flexibility of movement, the other hand (or in the case of a double amputee, the other terminal) can be used to make further adjustments, such as twisting the wrist into 12 different positions.*

For general use, the artificial hand (above inset) gives a firm prehensile grip between the thumb and the index and middle fingers. The third and little fingers follow the movement of the other fingers and are spring-loaded to accommodate the shape of whatever is being grasped. There are two types of body-powered hands: voluntary open (VO), in which the hand is opened with the cable and closes automatically; and voluntary close (VC), in which the hand closes when tension is applied to the cable.

A wide variety of terminal attachments are available for specific purposes, including grippers and holders for mechanic and carpentry tools, eating utensils, and outdoor recreation devices. When the hand is in use, a cosmetic silicone glove can be worn, which has a realistic color and texture matching the wearer's natural skin tone. The glove is also stain-resistant and can be extended to midway up the forearm.

Questions and Answers

I have been told that I have a malignant tumor in my breast and I am due to have a mastectomy. Is it possible to have an internal breast prosthesis put in at the same time as the mastectomy?

Yes. Some surgeons will be willing to do this at the same time as a mastectomy. The surgeon will try to remove as little breast tissue as possible, and to leave the skin intact. He or she will then restore the normal contours of the breast by the insertion of an implant. However, if you decide to wait a while for more surgery the surgeon will leave more skin behind than usual, and you can wear an external prosthesis until you have the implant inserted.

How soon after I have my mastectomy will I be able to wear an external prosthesis?

It can be worn almost immediately, but most surgeons wait until the stitches have been removed before recommending its use. The prosthesis is fitted into the bra and can easily be worn over the wound before it has fully healed.

After a leg has been amputated, is it always possible for a prosthesis to be fitted?

A functioning prosthesis, on which the patient is able to bear weight, can be used as soon as the stump has healed. However, this period of time can sometimes be prolonged, especially if the amputation was performed for poor blood supply. The final result in terms of walking depends on the overall physical condition of the patient and the level of the amputation, together with his or her mental attitude toward wanting to walk again.

My wife has had an artificial heart valve for five years now. How long is it likely to last? Will it wear out?

It should last for many more years. Fully artificial heart valves made from plastic will last longer than pig heart valves.

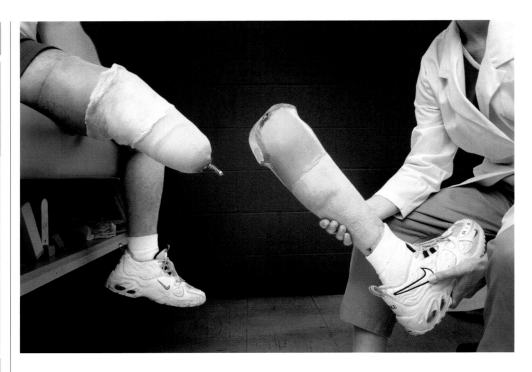

▲ *When a person loses a leg, he or she will be fitted with an artificial (prosthetic) limb. The limb has a reflex foot action and a high activity knee module. At the top is the colored upper leg support and brace. The knee module contains a piston that absorbs pressure from the leg as the knee bends. The foot moves by reflex action in relation to the leg using a spring-loaded mechanism. The foot absorbs the weight of the body and moves synchronously with the action of the leg.*

the patient's stump, the more control he or she will have over the prosthesis. Most artificial legs are held in place with a combination of straps and a slight suction effect caused by the stump's sitting in a bucket-shaped recess at the top of the prosthesis. A patient who is otherwise well soon learns to control the prosthesis and, with the help of physical therapy, gradually regains strength in the muscles in the remaining part of the limb.

The materials used for making these prostheses are a combination of metal, plastic, and leather; most artificial limbs are custom-made for the patient.

Arms

Whereas the lower limb prosthesis involves bearing the weight of the body, the prosthesis for the upper limb involves far more subtle functions. The hand is such a complex and versatile part of the body that replacement of it by artificial means is a delicate process (see Hand). Trials are ongoing to improve upper limb prostheses with a functioning hand, and it is likely that further advances in technology will happen. Certain prostheses have been developed that can be attached to existing muscles in the stump so that movement is controlled by the brain. There are limbs available with joints powered by gas pressure that can perform many functions of grasping and manipulation. The thalidomide tragedy has probably acted as a stimulus because its victims were born without arms. Victims often had hands attached directly to their shoulders, so a prosthesis can be manipulated at the top end by the patients' fingers, giving them a much better functional result than patients who have had to have their arms amputated (see Thalidomide). New technology has improved the appearance if not the functioning of prostheses; skin with a very lifelike appearance has been created with creases, pores, and fingerprints, and like human skin, with three skin layers.

Joint prostheses

Arthritis (inflammation of joints) is a common disease. Until the introduction of joint replacement, arthritis could usually be treated only with drugs and with physical therapy. Nowadays there are many joints that can be replaced (see Joints). The most common and, as yet, most successful is hip joint replacement, but there are also operations to replace the knee joint,

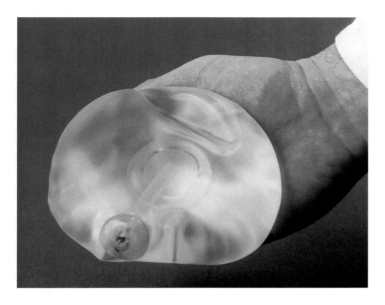

▲ *A wide variety of breast prostheses are available for women who have had to undergo a mastectomy (breast removal). These prostheses are often made from silicone and can be closely matched in size, consistency, and weight to a woman's natural breast.*

shoulder joint, elbow joint, and small joints in the fingers. A patient who has a hip joint prosthesis is often converted from being an invalid to being as active an individual as he or she was before. Pain, which is a characteristic feature of arthritis, is completely abolished, and often the range of movement at the joint is greatly improved. Even though it is a major operation, the patient usually recovers quickly. He or she is usually up and walking a few days after surgery and is often home after a week or 10 days. When the wound has healed and the strength in the muscles has been built up, there is often no further requirement for walking aids.

However, there are several problems inherent in replacing a joint. First, the materials used must be biologically inert. That is, they must not cause a reaction in the tissues, and they must not corrode over the years. Second, they must be strong enough to withstand many years of wear and tear. Third, there has to be some way of fixing the two parts of the joint to the bones which make up the joint. After many years of research, the best combination has been found to be a metal ball fitting into a plastic socket. The two components are then fixed to the bone using a special acrylic cement.

Another problem associated with implanting artificial joints into the body is infection. If infection takes hold in the region of the artificial material, then it is virtually impossible to get rid of the infection until the material has been removed. Although extreme care with technique, together with the use of antibiotics at the time of surgery, has helped to reduce the incidence of infection to a very low level, it does still occur (see Antibiotics; Infection and Infectious Diseases).

Heart valves

Since the advent of open-heart surgery in the early 1950s, there have been many designs for prosthetic heart valves. The normal valves in the heart consist of two or three main sheets of fibrous material, which are attached to the inside of the heart and are designed so that they snap together when blood tries to flow in the wrong direction. When blood flows in the right direction, they are pressed back against the sides of the heart, allowing the blood to flow with no resistance (see Heart). When the valves are diseased, either they become thickened so that there is an increase in resistance to flow, or they become weak, so that the blood can leak through them.

The most common types of prosthetic valves in use today are the Starr valve and the Bjorle-Shiley valve. The Starr valve consists of a metal cage inside which is a plastic ball. The metal cage has a ring at one end and this ring is stitched to the inside of the heart. The ball can move about inside the cage, but as soon as it lodges in the ring, the blood cannot flow through. Therefore, it allows blood to flow in one direction only. The Bjorle-Shiley valve has a similar ring, which is stitched to the inside of the heart. In the ring is a tiny trapdoor which can open and close. Again, the blood is able to flow in only one direction.

The main problems associated with these valves are that blood can clot on the foreign material, and that the constant movement of the valve can damage the red blood cells, leading to anemia. The

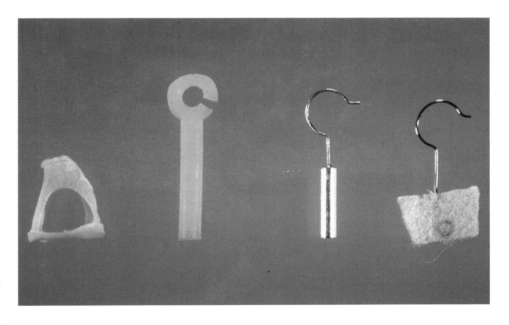

▲ *Sound is transmitted from the eardrum to the inner ear via a chain of three tiny movable bones, one of which is called the stapes bone. If this bony chain becomes fused or rigid as the result of disease, it can be remobilized by means of a prosthetic stapes, which will greatly increase the patient's level of hearing. However, stapedectomies are not suitable to treat deafness that has been caused by disease or damage to the nerve carrying impulses to the brain. This photograph shows the natural human stapes bone (left); a Teflon stapes (second from left); and two different types of metal stapes.*

STAPEDECTOMY

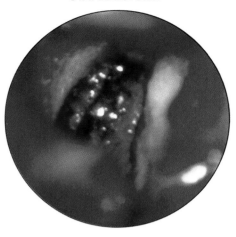

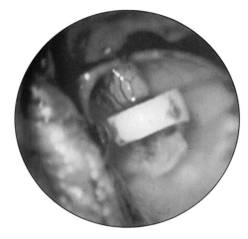

▲ *To insert a prosthetic Teflon stapes, the natural bone is first removed.*

▲ *A platform is then prepared for the Teflon replacement.*

▲ *The prosthetic stapes is then inserted into the middle ear.*

former problem can be dealt with by giving the patient special drugs to prevent the blood from clotting; the latter, if it does cause a significant loss of red blood cells, has to be treated by giving the patient a blood transfusion.

Breast prostheses

Breast prostheses have been used for many years (see Breasts). They are usually used to increase the size of the breasts in patients who have small breasts. These patients are either those whose breasts have failed to develop, or those whose breasts have been greatly reduced in size following childbirth and lactation (see Breast-Feeding; Lactation). Breast prostheses can be used after a mastectomy.

The material must have several characteristics to be successful. First, like any other substance implanted in the body, it has to be biologically inert; second, it has to have the same consistency as breast tissue; and third, it has to maintain this consistency for many years. The material that is most popular now is saline, in the form of a bag of jellylike fluid. Because its shape can be altered, it can be inserted through an incision on the undersurface of the existing breast, and is placed in the space between the muscles of the chest wall and the existing breast. The prostheses are manufactured in various sizes, and the most suitable size is chosen. The operation is a great success provided that infection is not a problem. If an infection does occur, the prosthesis usually has to be removed.

The use of these prostheses after surgery for cancer of the breast is no longer a matter for argument. There is no evidence that the patient is at risk of developing a further tumor, and the presence of a prosthesis does not interfere with a breast examination, because it goes underneath the woman's own tissue and chest muscles. Therefore, it does not affect the ability of the doctor to assess whether a recurrence of the tumor has in fact taken place (see Cancer; Tumors).

External breast prostheses, which are also made of a bag containing fluid or gel, are in general use after a mastectomy. With careful attention, many women are able to disguise completely the fact that they have had a mastectomy.

In the ear

Sound that enters the ear impinges on the eardrum. In turn, this is conveyed to the inner ear via a chain of tiny bones, where the sound is converted into nervous impulses. In the disease otosclerosis, the inner of the three bones, the stapes, becomes fused into the wall of the inner ear, diminishing the amount of sound transmitted. The diseased bone can be removed and a small plastic or metal one substituted, with a dramatic increase in the level of hearing. The advantage here is that the prosthesis is in the air-containing middle ear, acting like a bridge between the eardrum and the inner ear, and so is not enclosed in tissue which could otherwise react with it (see Hearing).

The male genitalia

When a testis has to be removed because of injury, tumor, or twisting, a prosthetic testis made of plastic can be inserted. The operation is sometimes done at the time of removal of the testis, but it can also be done later, particularly if there is any inflammation.

Various diseases of the penis can also be helped by prostheses (see Penis and Disorders). There is a disease, called priapism, in which the patient develops a painful erection caused by a thrombosis of the veins leading away from the penis (see Erection and Ejaculation; Thrombosis). When the condition is resolved, the patient is sometimes left with an inability to obtain an erection. Insertion of a silastic prosthesis into the shaft of the penis enables the patient to penetrate the vagina during sexual intercourse and possibly to maintain fertility.

The future

The field of prosthetics is wide open to new developments. Stronger and lighter materials such as Vitallium, titanium, and harder plastics are being created, and electronic technology will further the development of functional prostheses such as the hand (see Medical Research).

See also: **Arthritis; Artificial limbs; Deafness; Hip; Joint replacement; Mastectomy; Open-heart surgery; Physical therapy; Surgery; Testes**

Protein

Questions and Answers

What happens if you don't eat any protein?

Protein is an essential part of the diet. If people are starving, they usually do not have enough protein or energy-producing food, so the body breaks down its own protein to act as a fuel, losing much muscle bulk. Lack of protein in a normal-calorie diet leads to a condition called kwashiorkor, which mainly occurs in young children.

Is too much protein bad for you?

Normally, the body metabolizes excess protein to produce energy. Protein imbalances in the body can be a sign of disease. Some tumors produce antibodies, increasing the globulin level in the blood. In conditions such as meningitis, protein levels around the brain and spinal cord are raised. Kidney failure can allow albumin from the bloodstream to leak away.

My father has kidney failure and the doctors have put him on a low-protein diet. Why?

One of the tasks of the kidneys is to remove waste products, many of which result from the body's use of protein. The main waste product is urea, which is formed as a result of protein breakdown. If the protein level is kept low in the diet of someone with failing kidneys, less urea is produced, so that there is less work for the kidneys to do.

Is protein the best sort of food to eat if you want to put on weight and build yourself up?

If you actually want to build up your body's muscle content and strength, the way to do it is by exercise that encourages the muscles to grow. Just eating more protein without any exercise, however, would simply be an expensive way of putting on fat.

Most people think of protein simply as an important part of the diet. In fact, everything from the color of the hair to inherited talents is determined by the way people's bodies are genetically programmed to make proteins.

The three main classes of food are proteins, fats, and carbohydrates. Fats and carbohydrates supply our energy needs, while proteins are the actual building blocks from which the body is made. A minimum intake is needed to maintain the body's reconstruction and repair processes so that it remains healthy, especially in growing children (see Growth).

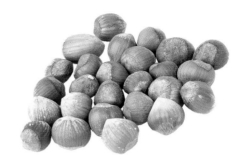

What is protein?

Protein molecules are twisted chains of smaller compounds called amino acids, which are vital to the body's survival. Proteins are the only major food group to contain nitrogen. Twenty amino acids make up all the proteins found in food; eight are essential to the diet, since the body cannot make them itself. The other 12 can be made in the body, although its ability to do this sometimes fails. Acids and enzymes in the digestive system break down food protein into its constituent amino acids. These can then be absorbed by the intestine, passed on to the liver, and enter the bloodstream.

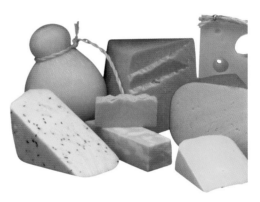

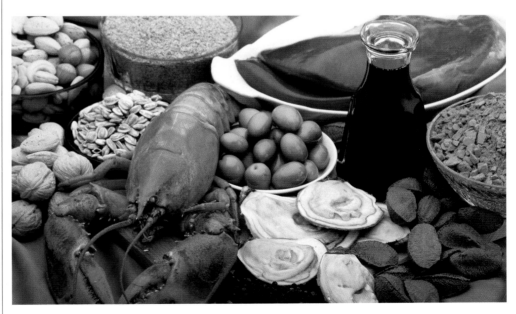

▲ *These foods contain relatively high amounts of protein. Cheese contains about 0.88 oz. (25 g) of protein in every 3.5 oz. (100 g) of weight. Prime beef contains 0.75 oz. (21 g). Proteins in nuts range from almonds at 0.65 oz. (18.6 g) to hazelnuts (top photo) at 0.44 oz. (12.6 g). Oysters, although still high in protein, contain only 0.29 oz. (8.2 g).*

STRUCTURE OF PROTEIN

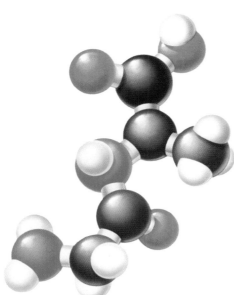

▼ *Protein chains are linked to parallel chains or are coiled around themselves to give the more complex secondary structure. The regularly wound coils of a helix (a spiral staircase shape) shown below are held in place by bonds (dotted lines) linking the oxygen and hydrogen atoms in different amino acids. Each amino acid also has a side chain called R (purple); the constituents of the R chain vary according to the individual amino acid.*

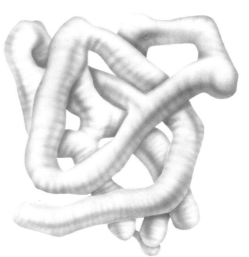

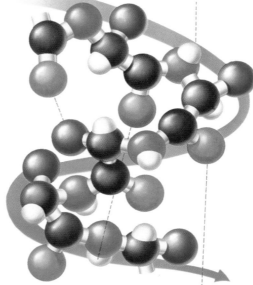

▲ *Proteins are composed of chains of amino acid molecules, each of which is made up of atoms of carbon (black), hydrogen (white), oxygen (red), and nitrogen (blue). There are 20 different amino acids generally found in proteins. The number of amino acids, and the order in which they are arranged in a particular protein chain, make up the primary structure of proteins. Shown above are two amino acids linked in a protein chain.*

▲ *The third structure of a protein concerns its overall three-dimensional shape. Some proteins, including the enzymes, are curled around themselves into entwined knots to give a globular shape. However, there is a great variety and range of proteins according to their composition, size, and shape—those which have a purely structural function (the building blocks) are less convoluted than the enzyme above.*

Although tissues such as the liver can store some amino acids taken into the body after a protein meal, the body has no major store of protein or amino acids. Fat and carbohydrate, in contrast, can both be stored in large quantities.

What does protein do?

The most important role of protein within the body is as a building block. People's tissues are made with protein, and the central substance of connective tissues holding the various organs and tissues together is a protein molecule called collagen.

Enzymes are also protein molecules. They act as catalysts for the chemical reactions the body depends upon. Proteins also circulate in the blood. The small molecules of albumin help keep fluid in the bloodstream; the larger group of globulin proteins includes the immunoglobulins or antibodies, the body's main defense against infection (see Blood; Immune System).

Some hormones are proteins, and they are also vital to the overall functioning of the body. Insulin is an example of a protein hormone;

it is made of two protein chains linked together (see Insulin). The body's entire protein structure is renewed about once every 60 days. Food and recycled body proteins replenish the blood, liver, and other tissues, and cells drain this supply to make new proteins.

Protein and genetics

Heredity is based on a code passed from one generation to the next, telling the cells how to make proteins. Information in the chromosomes specifies the amino acid sequence in each body protein. Every inherited characteristic, from eye color to musical talent, originates in coded instructions passed on by the parents. As far as scientists know, these coded instructions concern only the way in which cells are told to make proteins (see Heredity).

See also: **Cells and chromosomes; Diet; Digestive system; Enzymes; Fats; Genetics; Hormones; Kidneys and kidney diseases; Metabolism; Muscles**

Protozoal infections

Questions and Answers

In Guatemala I met someone with "espundia"; he had severe facial disfigurement from loss of tissue. Could I have caught the disease?

Espundia is a form of the protozoal disease leishmaniasis that is transmitted by the bite of the sand fly. Although you may have been bitten by sand flies it is unlikely that you will get cutaneous leishmaniasis. The symptoms are one or more painless skin nodules that are slow to heal, and diagnosis can be made by microscopic examination of material from the nodules. Treatment may be unnecessary.

My gynecologist says that my vaginal irritation is caused by a trichomonal infection. Could I have infected my partner?

Vaginal trichomoniasis is caused by the flagellated protozoon *Trichomonas vaginalis*. While this occurs commonly in the vagina, it may also infect the urethra or the prostate gland in men, and you probably acquired it from a sexual partner. Your partner is likely to be infected, so it is essential that both of you are treated. The drug metronidazole (Flagyl) is effective.

A friend died from a strange infection called balamuthia, for which there is no treatment. Is it a common disease? Could I get it?

It is a rare infection by an amoeba called *Balamuthia mandrillaris* first described in 1990. Balamuthia causes a brain inflammation that can affect humans and animals. The body responds to the infection by producing masses of cells and small blood vessels, called granulation tissue, in the brain and on the face. There is no known effective treatment. Your friend may have caught the infection from an animal, but it is most unlikely that you will get the disease.

With one or two minor exceptions, protozoal infections are relatively rare in the United States. However, in less developed countries certain protozoa, such as the parasites that are responsible for malaria, affect millions of people and are responsible for ill health and many deaths.

Protozoa are simple, single-cell organisms, larger and more complex than bacteria, that form a subkingdom of the animal kingdom. They differ from all other animals in that, as cells, they remain separate from each other and do not join up permanently to form tissues. A single individual is called a protozoon or protozoan. The name derives from the Greek *proto*, meaning "first" and *zoon*, meaning "animal."

Mobility

The range of protozoa is enormous and includes many different classes and species. Although only a small proportion of protozoa actually cause disease, in the developing world protozoal disease is one of the important causes of serious ill health.

Protozoa are complex organisms, and most are capable of movement. Some move by means of a long, whiplike filament called a flagellum; others are covered with fine, rapidly lashing, hairlike processes called cilia that allow rapid movement. Many are amoebic and move by pushing out a bulge called a pseudopodium and then flowing into it.

Method of spread

Like all single-cell organisms, protozoa can survive only in a liquid environment, so many of those that cause disease are acquired as waterborne infections. Food can be contaminated by parasites following infection with fecal matter by food handlers. Being microscopic, however, protozoa survive well in a very thin film of fluid and can be transmitted by contact with body fluids as in

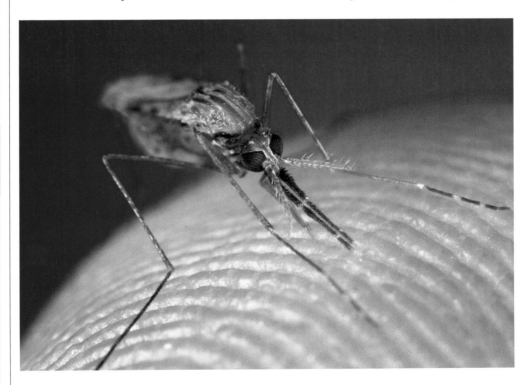

▲ *A female mosquito,* Anopheles gambiae, *feeds on human flesh.*

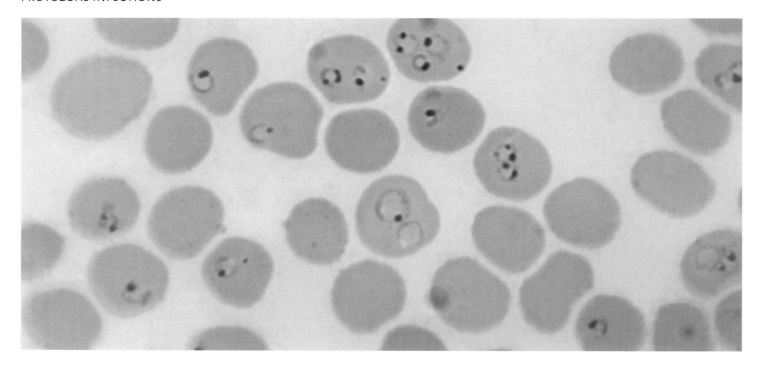

▲ *A photomicrograph of a blood smear showing rings of* **Plasmodium falciparum** *in the red cells. This is the parasite that causes malaria in humans.*

some sexually transmitted species such as *Trichomonas* and *Giardia*. The most important disease-producing protozoan of all, however, is the malarial parasite, which is transmitted by being carried from person to person by a bite from a female anopheline mosquito. Leishmaniasis, another important protozoal infection, is spread by the bite of a sand fly.

Malaria

The name of this disease arose from the Italian *mala*, meaning "bad"; and *aria*, meaning "air," before the true cause was known. Malaria is responsible for at least one million deaths each year throughout the world, and is caused by one of several different species of protozoal parasites of the genus *Plasmodium*. The protozoa undergo breeding cycles in the blood; but once the illness is over, breeding cycles in the liver can cause further attacks months or years later as the liver protozoa break out into the blood.

Heavy infection can be very dangerous for two reasons. The protozoa can block the small blood vessels of the brain and cause dangerous and often fatal cerebral malaria. They can also rupture so many of the red blood cells that the released hemoglobin colors the urine dark red or black. This is called blackwater fever, and the destruction of blood cells causes dangerous anemia.

Amebiasis

Another important protozoal disease is caused by the amoeba, *Entamoeba histolytica*. This is an active tissue-destroying parasite that leads to widespread damage of the large intestine (amebic dysentery), and sometimes abscesses in the liver, lungs, and brain. Amebic dysentery is an acute, inflammatory infection of the colon caused by the burrowing of an amoeba into the inner coat of the bowel, causing ulceration with pain and diarrhea. The amoebae undermine the bowel lining and enter the veins in the wall of the intestine. They are then carried to the liver, where they are capable of causing large abscesses.

Trypanosomiasis

African trypanosomiasis is a disease of the nervous system known as sleeping sickness. The disease is caused by a *Trypanosoma* protozoan. The symptoms are extensive brain inflammation causing headache, sleepiness, lassitude, a vacant expression, drooping eyelids, and finally loss of all motivation so that the affected person may starve to death. South American trypanosomiasis, also known as Chagas' disease, is spread by a painless bite from the cone-nosed or assassin bug. In endemic areas, Chagas' disease is a major cause of heart damage and heart failure.

Other protozoal diseases

Other diseases caused by protozoa include leishmaniasis, which may seriously affect the internal organs (kala-azar), or the skin (cutaneous leishmaniasis); and giardiasis, an intestinal infection with the protozoan *Giardia lamblia*, which is usually acquired in contaminated drinking water but is also transmitted sexually, and which causes diarrhea with flatulence, cramping, and abdominal pain. Protozoa cause a vaginal infection trichomonal vaginitis; cryptosporidiosis, a common cause of travelers' diarrhea, which may be very dangerous to people with immune deficiency; balantidiasis, which causes a type of dysentery with large ulcers in the lining of the colon; isosporiasis, which most commonly affects people with AIDS; and microsporidiosis, an infection caused by various protozoal organisms of the genus *Microsporidia*, which can also cause serious corneal infections and ulceration. *Acanthamoeba polyphaga* is an amoebic protozoan that can affect the eyes, especially of people who wear contact lenses.

See also: **Infection and infectious diseases; Malaria; Parasites; Trichomoniasis**

Psittacosis

Questions and Answers

Is it true you can catch psittacosis only from parrots, or can you get it from any type of bird?

The main sources of psittacosis are parrots, but many species of bird can be carriers of the disease. In the United States, parrots and pigeons are the main sources.

If I buy a parrot, how can I be sure to get one free of psittacosis?

First, check that the bird appears healthy, with nice shiny feathers. However, even if the bird looks and seems healthy, it could still be carrying the disease. Rely on the reputation of the dealer. Make sure that his or her premises are clean and hygienic and the cages are not overcrowded. Also, check that the bird has been bred in this country and has not just been brought in from abroad.

How could I tell if my parrot was about to get psittacosis?

The disease is common in parrots and is endemic in most aviaries. Many birds carry the disease without showing any symptoms; these tend to appear with any form of stress, such as overcrowding. Infection is less likely to cause trouble with a single pet at home, but can still lead to disease in humans. An infected bird will become listless and its abdomen will be distended. There is often diarrhea. You must avoid contact with the bird, and a veterinarian should put it to sleep immediately.

Do people die from psittacosis?

Psittacosis is rarely fatal. More often it causes a flulike illness. Without proper treatment, it can cause prolonged pneumonia. Occasionally, the organism can infect the heart valves, and this infection does lead to a more serious illness.

People who keep birds as pets run the risk of developing psittacosis, which is an infectious disease caused by the bacterium *Chlamydia psittaci*. It causes symptoms similar to pneumonia, accompanied by high fever.

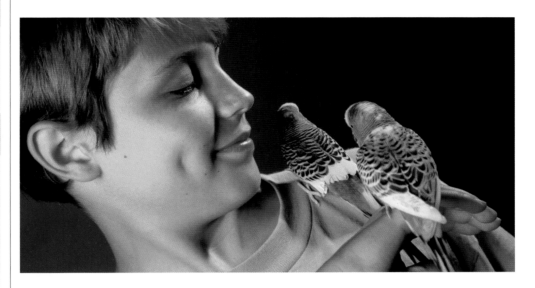

▲ *People who have daily contact with birds may be at risk of psittacosis.*

The parrot family are called psittacines, and psittacosis got its peculiar name from that term. However, the disease can also occur in pigeons, turkeys, ducks, and geese.

Psittacosis is caused by the bacterial parasite *Chlamydia psittaci*, which can be transmitted from birds to humans (see Parasites). People usually contract the disease by inhaling dust particles contaminated with the excrement of infected birds. Only about 150 cases are reported each year, but because the illness can be similar to flu, some cases are never recognized (see Influenza).

People who own a single, caged bird are not very likely to catch the disease, but bird breeders are especially vulnerable. The disease is usually found in aviaries, where birds may start showing symptoms if they are under stress, for example, from overcrowded cages or the arrival of new birds.

Symptoms and dangers

Psittacosis may seem similar to influenza. What distinguishes it is that the patient's lungs are always affected. If a chest X ray is taken, large shadows appear, indicating infection. This may last for some time after the illness has improved. Severe headache is also common. If the symptoms are left untreated, the patient can develop prolonged pneumonia.

Patients with the disease usually tell the doctor they have been exposed to birds, and the diagnosis becomes more likely if one of the birds has become sick. A blood test is usually performed because, as with any other infection, patients will form antibodies to the organism, which show up in blood. Psittacosis itself is not a very dangerous disease, although deaths have been recorded. Occasionally, patients may get the infection in their heart valves, or even the brain, and then a serious illness may occur, which may be a threat to life.

Treatment and outlook

Most patients recover without treatment but, if needed, the antibiotic tetracycline or penicillin may be given. However, this must be given early in the illness to be effective, whereas diagnosis is not often made until a later stage.

> **See also:** Antibiotics; Bacteria; Hygiene; Infection and infectious diseases; Lung and lung disorders; Penicillin; Pneumonia; Tetracyclines

Psoriasis

I have recurring psoriasis, and recently my scalp has become scaly. At first I thought I had dandruff, but could I have psoriasis?

Yes. Psoriasis often spreads to the scalp. It can be treated with medicated lotions such as corticosteroid preparations; coal-tar shampoo can then be used to prevent the buildup of scale.

Are corticosteroid ointments for the skin dangerous?

No. When they were first produced in the 1960s, corticosteroid preparations were widely used with excellent results, but further treatment was usually needed for relapses. Over the years, the skin can become thin and inelastic, prone to infection, and less able to heal. Occasionally, the strongest preparations also produced side effects. However, the safe limits for prescribing corticosteroids are now recognized, and their use is restricted so that the patient does not suffer dangerous side effects.

Does sunlight help treat psoriasis?

Yes, except in rare cases. Ultraviolet light has been in use for some time as a treatment and is part of a treatment called PUVA. A psoralen (P) drug is given to sensitize the skin to sunlight; the skin is then irradiated with long-wave ultraviolet light (UVA). Although the skin clears up after treatment, relapse is common.

My doctor said I had eczema, but now says it is psoriasis. Why?

Eczema and psoriasis of the scalp and hands may alternate, but because the treatment differs it is important to distinguish between them. This can be done by examining other areas of the body where the symptoms will be much easier to diagnose.

Psoriasis is a common skin complaint that usually occurs in a mild form. Only rarely is it dangerous, and there are many different treatments that have been found to control the condition.

In psoriasis, the skin forms pink to dull red patches covered with characteristic silvery white scaling. It is usually a chronic condition with acute phases of eruption followed by remissions.

Causes

The underlying cause of psoriasis is that new skin cells are produced about 10 times faster than normal (see Cells and Chromosomes). As a result, the cells accumulate and form thickened patches covered with dead, flaking skin.

There is much evidence to suggest a genetic inheritance of the disease, and it is often the case that a newly diagnosed psoriasis sufferer finds that a relative may also have the condition (see Genetic Diseases and Disorders: Genetics; Heredity).

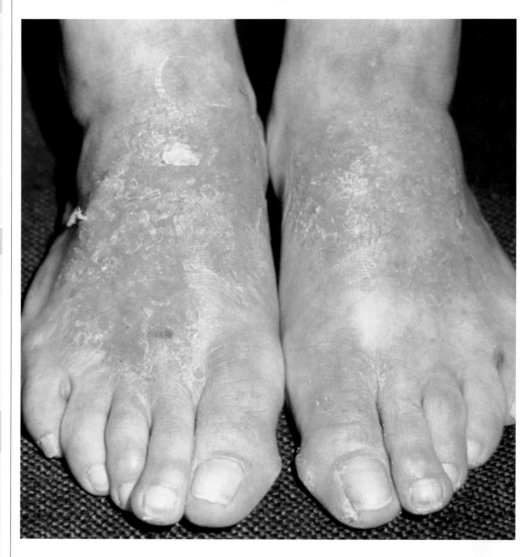

▲ *Scaly patches on the skin that cause irritation are typical of psoriasis, even in this mild case of a relatively rare type known as guttate psoriasis.*

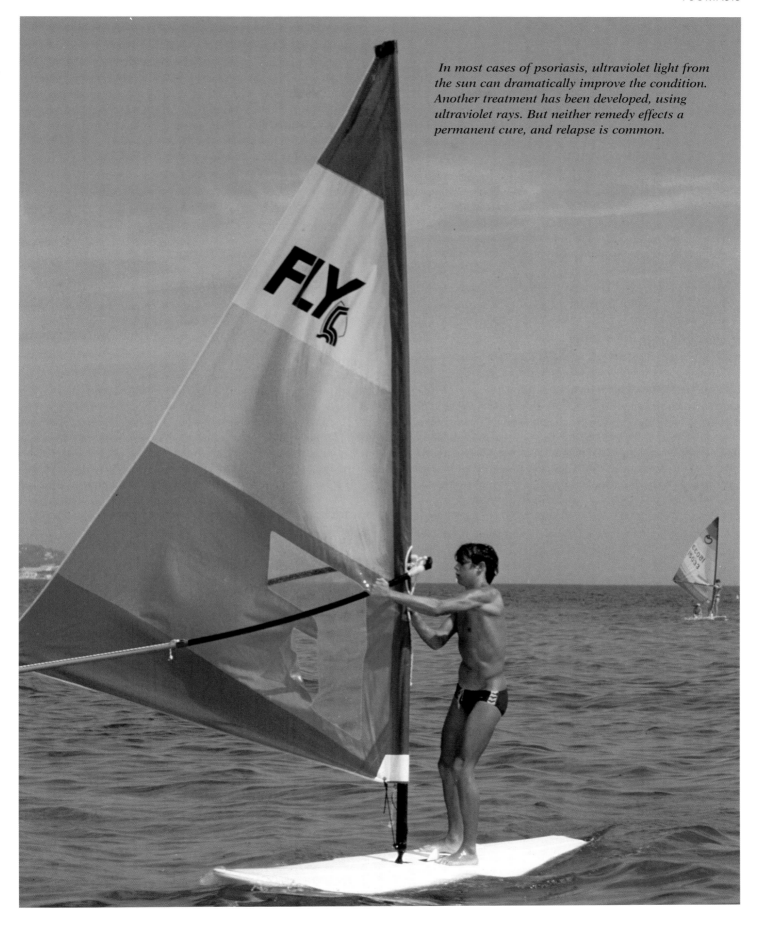

In most cases of psoriasis, ultraviolet light from the sun can dramatically improve the condition. Another treatment has been developed, using ultraviolet rays. But neither remedy effects a permanent cure, and relapse is common.

There are many things that can trigger psoriasis. Physical and chemical trauma can precipitate it, and when it occurs in already damaged skin it is called the Koebner phenomenon. A general infection such as influenza may also trigger a relapse of the disease.

Hormonal changes seem to influence the incidence of psoriasis in that it tends to coincide with puberty and menopause (see Hormones). On the other hand, there is often a remission during pregnancy, with a relapse once the pregnancy is over. Drugs are rarely a precipitating factor, although an association has been noted with certain drugs used to treat malaria.

Psychological causes are of variable importance in psoriasis. It may be triggered by an emotionally stressful event such as an examination or bereavement (see Stress), and some studies by psychiatrists indicate that psoriasis may be an outward expression of subconscious problems (see Psychosomatic Problems). Understanding and resolution of conflicts may help to improve psoriasis.

Incidence
According to the statistics for 2003 compiled by the National Psoriasis Foundation, psoriasis occurs in about 2.1 percent of the population of the United States. It occurs in both sexes, but is slightly more prevalent in women. The condition usually appears between the ages of 15 and 35, but it can develop at any age (10 to 15 percent of sufferers develop it before the age of 10).

Symptoms and types
The scaly patches that form during psoriasis tend to persist and may coalesce. The skin gets thicker, and the silvery white scale builds up and becomes flaky. There is no pain, but there may be irritation. The skin does not bleed unless the surface is damaged by scratching. If the scale is peeled off, many tiny bleeding points can be seen where the blood vessels run up into the thickened skin.

There are few symptoms in psoriasis, but other conditions are sometimes associated with it. It is sometimes accompanied by a painful swelling and stiffness of the joints (see Arthritis). The nails may also become thickened, pitted, or separated from their beds (see Nails).

There are many types of psoriasis. The most common is the appearance of plaques (patches of erupted skin) from one to several inches across. This is called plaque psoriasis, or by its scientific name psoriasis vulgaris, and can affect any part of the body, but especially the knees, legs, elbows, scalp, and genitals.

Children—and, occasionally, adults—may get another type, called guttate psoriasis, in which showers of little red psoriasis spots appear on the trunk, upper arms, upper legs, face, genitals, feet, and scalp. This is an uncommon form of the disease and usually occurs after an ear or throat infection.

Flexural psoriasis occurs in the flexures (creases) of the armpits and groin. There is no scaling and all that is visible is a red patch. This may be confused with a fungal infection, but the distinction is that a fungal infection is red at the edges, whereas psoriatic skin is uniformly red all over.

A rare and more serious form is pustular psoriasis, in which the skin erupts in pus-filled spots (see Pus). These are sterile and are due to an inflammatory response in the skin. When this kind of psoriasis is restricted to the hands and feet it remains harmless, although it may be difficult to treat. However, generalized pustular psoriasis, in which the skin all over the body erupts in these pus-filled spots, is a dangerous condition needing hospital treatment.

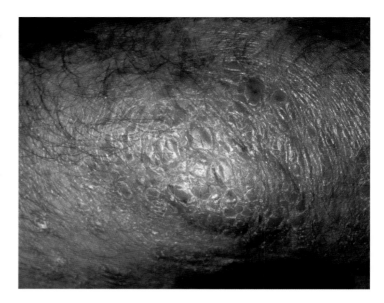

▲ *The arm of a patient shows the thick, dry, silvery plaques on the elbow that are the main symptom of plaque psoriasis.*

Treatment
Treatment of psoriasis consists of lifestyle and medical measures. After it has been diagnosed, a patient may have to adjust his or her life to cope with the disease. Some people may need to change their job if substances that they deal with irritate the skin (see Occupational Hazards). In any case, time must be taken off work to rest during flare-ups.

Psoriasis of the hands and feet may be difficult to diagnose. The scaling may look like eczema, and the natural thickness of the skin may mask the other signs of the disease (see Eczema). Often, only its presence elsewhere in the body finally clinches the diagnosis.

The basis of medical treatment is direct application of medication onto the diseased skin. In the acute phase of eruption only bland preparations like weak corticosteroid ointment and salicylic acid are used (see Steroids). Once the skin settles down, much stronger substances are needed to remove the thick scale that remains. The drug dithranol, various coal-tar preparations, mild steroid creams, and ultraviolet light are the mainstays of treatment.

However, coal-tar preparations are usually too strong for the scalp, face, genitals, and flexures, so here corticosteroid ointments are often used in differing strengths. These slow the psoriatic process but do not cure it. However, they are very useful when other treatments are unsuccessful and may also be prescribed for difficult areas such as hands.

Stronger remedies are available for resistant cases, including the use of ultraviolet light. A doctor should be consulted further if a problem such as an uncontrolled flare-up occurs.

Outlook
Although psoriasis tends to recur, most psoriasis sufferers will get to know what preparation suits their skin best in treating the complaint. People who can also learn to tolerate the discomfort of the condition are at a great advantage.

See also: **Hair and scalp disorders; Skin and skin diseases**

Psychiatry

Questions and Answers

Is there any truth in the saying that genius is next to madness?

Not exactly, but there are several reasons why this idea should have developed. Even if someone has a major psychiatric disorder, such as schizophrenia, only a small part of the brain function is disordered. Even if a psychiatric disorder causes people to believe, for example, that they are being followed or spied on, it may not have any other effect on thoughts, and feelings and knowledge may be unaffected. Vincent van Gogh produced beautiful work while suffering from a psychiatric disorder, as did the composer Robert Schumann. A person with a psychiatric disorder, just like a person with asthma, may be a brilliant lawyer or doctor, or an underachiever. Clever, original thinkers may be regarded as mentally ill when they are merely eccentric. Original thinkers like Galileo or Darwin may be considered mentally ill because their ideas threaten established belief.

Are psychiatric disorders infectious?

One very rare form of degenerative psychiatric disorder is caused by an infective agent called a prion. This is Creutzfeldt-Jakob disease; its effects are more physical then psychiatric. Some diseases that can cause brain damage are infectious. They include various forms of meningitis, and syphilis, which can cause brain damage many years later if left untreated.

My brother is to be discharged from a psychiatric unit: is it likely that he will be dangerous?

It is very unlikely. No hospital would discharge such a patient. Immoral but psychiatrically well people are more likely to harm others than are mentally ill patients who have had therapy.

The practice of psychiatry does not have all the answers to emotional or psychiatric problems, but it has, in recent years, made great progress toward helping and curing those with psychological disorders.

Society's attitude toward people with psychiatric disorders has come a long way since the days when anyone emotionally disturbed was considered to be possessed by the devil. Psychiatry—a term derived from two Greek words meaning "mind" and "healing"—is a branch of medicine that specializes in the study, diagnosis, treatment, and prevention of psychiatric disorders.

In earlier times psychiatric disorders were assumed to be evidence of divine displeasure or manifestations of demonic possession. This attitude persisted until the 5th century B.C.E., when a Greek philosopher, Hippocrates, introduced a scientific approach to psychiatric disorders. He and

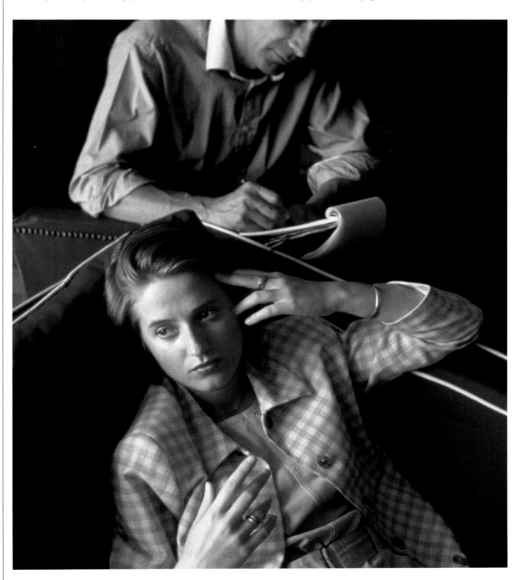

▲ *A psychiatrist will ask many questions about a patient's background and family in an attempt to diagnose the patient's problem. Once a diagnosis has been established, the psychiatrist may decide to treat the patient with drugs, or some type of therapy.*

Questions and Answers

Is there a danger of becoming addicted to drugs that are used to treat psychiatric disorders?

You can become dependent on almost any drug, even if it has no physically addictive properties. This is called psychological dependency. Also, all sleeping pills (hypnotics) and anxiety-reducing drugs can become mildly addictive if large doses are taken over a long period. Medications prescribed for the treatment of severe depression or problems such as schizophrenia or bipolar disorder are not addictive but are necessary to keep the illness at bay, much as insulin may be necessary to keep a diabetic patient stable.

Is it possible to recognize a psychiatric disorder in oneself and realize that a visit to a psychiatrist is necessary?

Yes. Many people ask for psychiatric help because of depression or anxiety and an inability to cope. They may want help with sleeping or to overcome a damaging habit. In more serious psychiatric illness, it can be difficult for victims to recognize the signs of the problem in themselves. However, some people with recurring psychiatric disorders can pick up warning signs, and avoid a relapse by seeking help.

My son has been bullied at elementary school and has become quiet and timid at home. Should I take him to a child psychiatrist?

You should of course ask your son's teachers what he does to attract the attention of the bullies. If his timid manner continues at home on weekends and during vacations, he may be having problems communicating with the family, so he cannot recharge his batteries at home. The best course is to ask your doctor to give you a referral to a child psychiatrist or a family psychiatrist.

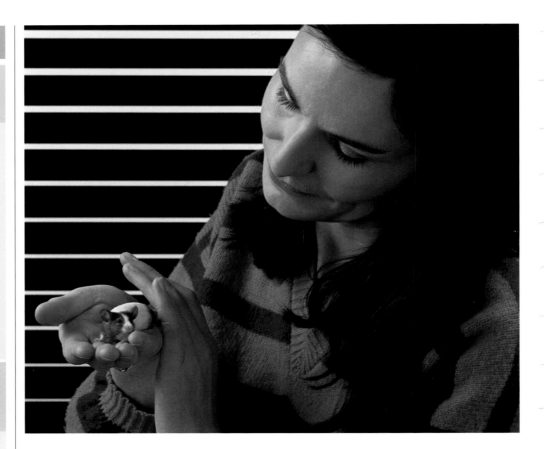

▲ *A phobia such as fear of mice may be gradually overcome by behavior therapy, in which the patient is brought to terms with the feared object.*

his successors were the first to describe and examine the clinical aspects of madness, and they laid the foundations for the science of psychiatry.

During medieval times, however, society's attitude toward psychiatric disorders regressed, and disorders of this kind were once again associated with witchcraft, demonic possession, and heresy. Even in the 16th and 17th centuries, while great advances were being made in physical medicine and surgery, psychiatric problems tended to be explained in terms of moral flaws and degeneration. In addition, it was common practice to confine the emotionally disturbed to institutions and madhouses, in which physical tortures were inflicted in the guise of treatment. It was a fashionable pastime in 17th-century London to take tours through the crowded cells of the Bedlam insane asylum and to watch the inmates tortured in public.

In the 19th century, conditions for people with psychiatric disorders improved, and scientific inquiry into the nature of insanity reemerged. Great strides were made in establishing a scientific basis for the study of psychiatric disorders, culminating in 1883 with a classification of disorders by Emil Kraepelin. Kraepelin was followed by Franz Mesmer, who used a form of hypnosis (which he called universal magnetic fluid) to treat disorders such as hysterical paralysis; Jean Martin Charcot, who placed hypnosis on a scientific basis; and Pierre Janet, who established a hierarchy of types of psychiatric function. This surge of inquiry into the nature of psychiatric disorders provided the background for Sigmund Freud to develop his psychoanalytic theory and practice.

Types of psychiatric problems

It has been claimed that 80 percent of women and 70 percent of men consult a doctor because of emotional difficulty at some time. Many people find it difficult to accept that they have emotional problems; they use minor physical ailments as the excuse for an appointment, but then they allude to underlying psychological ailments during the consultation.

Symptoms can range from mild, such as shyness in certain social situations, to severe, such as a feeling of near-suicidal helplessness all the time. Less commonly, some people have strange

Pioneers of modern psychiatry

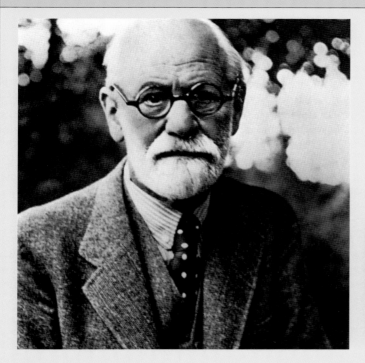

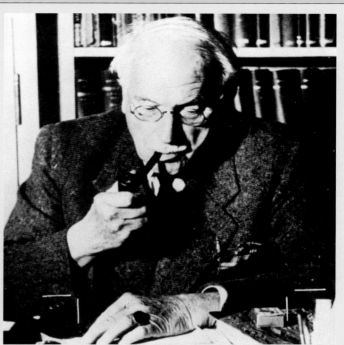

The foundations of psychoanalytic theory were laid by Sigmund Freud (above left). He introduced the technique of free association of ideas; patients are encouraged to say whatever comes into their minds, thus providing the analyst with valuable clues. Freud developed the study of the meaning of dreams, slips of the tongue, forgetfulness, and other mistakes and errors in everyday life. His researches led him to a new conception of the structure of personality, divided into the id, the inherited, instinctive impulses of the individual; the ego, the part of the mind that reacts to reality; and the superego, the part of the mind that exerts conscience and responds to social rule. He believed that anxiety arose from conflicts between these three facets of personality. Another of Freud's concepts, which he called transference, in which the analyst assumes the emotional status of a parent or lover, is said to be essential to the success of psychoanalysis. Finally, Freud created the libido theory of personality development as a psychosexual evolution that begins at birth and continues through childhood.

Carl Jung (above right) moved away from Freud's theories in an essentially mystical direction: whereas Freud used "libido" to describe sexual energy, Jung expanded its definition and linked it with what he called the collective unconscious, a reservoir of knowledge and experience.

Melanie Klein expanded the framework of psychoanalysis to include very young children. She claimed that their spontaneous play activities, utterances, and relationships with people around them could all be material for analysis.

experiences that other people do not share, such as hearing voices or music or seeing things.

While all psychiatric problems have the potential to interfere with normal life, some can scarcely be classed as illnesses, and these respond to simple help and guidance. Others fall into the category of diseases and may need urgent treatment, often with drugs and admittance to a psychiatric facility.

Just as there are separate floors in general hospitals for orthopedic or abdominal problems, many hospitals have separate units for psychiatric patients. Since psychiatric disorders are so common, there are also hospitals that specialize in psychiatric problems, just as certain hospitals specialize in eye disease.

Diagnosing psychiatric disorders

The psychiatrist's main diagnostic tool is simply listening to, and talking to, patients. He or she will want to know details about the patients' family background, family health, personalities, and interrelationships. He or she will also ask about patients' careers or jobs, about their health and feelings toward family and colleagues,

and about their sex life. Whatever information is filed by a psychiatrist will always remain confidential.

A lot of the information a psychiatrist asks for may seem irrelevant, but it is not. If, for example, a patient went to a doctor with pain in the left hand, and the doctor was allowed to examine only that part of the body, the diagnosis could be dangerously incomplete. The doctor would not be able to determine whether the cause of the pain was a coronary attack, pressure on the nerve roots, or an ailment of the limbs in general. In the same way, a psychiatrist has to obtain as complete a picture as possible of a patient's whole life, and the people in it; this will include information about past experiences and reactions.

Psychiatric treatment

Listening and talking are generally diagnostic tools, although treatment may also involve listening and talking. Once the patient's problem has been identified and isolated, many psychiatrists will prefer to use more physical methods of treatment, such as medicines and electroconvulsive therapy (ECT), or dynamic

Is it true that ECT can cause physical damage to the brain?

ECT (electroconvulsive therapy) produces temporary physical changes in the brain by the passage of an electrical current for a very brief time, and no permanent effects result unless the patient has something of the order of 80 or more sessions. Many highly intelligent people have had this treatment, and no impairment of their intellectual or other brain functions was found to follow.

My mother, age 74, is so confused that she is in a nursing home. Will the same thing necessarily happen to me?

The short answer is no. If your mother has some short-term or longer-term medical illness, such as stroke, thyroid trouble, or pernicious anemia, this may have led to her present confusion, and there is no reason to suspect a hereditary link in her psychiatric deterioration. If she has early Alzheimer's disease or dementia as a result of brain damage from a succession of silent strokes, the chance that you will develop the same condition is very slightly greater than if no one in your family was affected.

If I complain of depression to my doctor, will he try to eliminate any possible physical cause before giving me tranquilizers?

Your doctor will exclude the possibility of physical disease before treating you for depression. However, if you are young, are physically healthy, and have just had some obvious emotional upset like losing your job, he is less likely to carry out blood tests. If you are middle-aged and apparently secure, and the depression has come out of the blue, then he will give you a much more exhaustive examination. In any event he is more likely to give you antidepressants than tranquilizers, unless he thinks you are more worried than depressed.

techniques such as psychodrama or behavior therapy. As patients tell the psychiatrist about their early life or family, the psychiatrist will accumulate data concerning their state of mind, personality, and the people they turn to when in difficulty. Most patients will be quite frank in a general sense, but it is a characteristic of psychiatric disorders that, particularly in severe cases, patients cannot understand what is happening to them and cannot identify the source of turbulent feelings and thoughts.

One of the psychiatrist's most useful tools is the patient's body language. If the patient is depressed he or she may droop, speak slowly, and blink only rarely. An anxious person may sit on the edge of the chair, fidget with his or her fingers, sweat lightly, and speak in a quiet, high voice. Someone who feels angry or resentful tends to lean forward, juts out the chin, and speaks loudly. A patient suffering from hallucinations may pause to listen or look around for someone or something that is not there.

What a patient omits to say may help a psychiatrist: a trifling hesitation when mentioning a particular name, or a patient's attempts to avoid a subject such as extramarital sex, for example, can be vital clues to the patient's problem.

Physical health

A psychiatrist may require patients to undergo a thorough physical checkup. For instance, he or she may arrange tests for anemia, or tests to diagnose hormonal or glandular problems. Physical and psychiatric problems are often interconnected, and emotional tension often leads to bodily symptoms. Physical illness or trauma can induce psychological disturbances: many people experience depression after influenza, hepatitis, or pregnancy.

Psychiatrist: a doctor specializing in treatment of psychiatric disorders, and sometimes prescribing medicines

Psychologist: an expert on how the mind works, and ways to test it

Psychotherapist: a nonphysician therapist who treats patients by talking to them and listening to their problems

Psychoanalyst: a psychotherapist whose methods are based on the ideas of Freud and Jung, as well as other methods of psychotherapy

Behavior therapist: a psychiatrist, a psychologist, or a trained nurse who treats problems by training the patient to react in a different way

Counselor: often a nurse, or a lay-person with training, who advises on the practical approach to problems

Hypnotherapist: a therapist who uses hypnosis to relax patients and make them receptive to suggestions

Psychiatric nurse: a trained nurse who may visit and treat patients in their homes, as well as in the hospital

Specific psychiatric problems

There are three general categories of psychiatric disorders that psychiatrists often encounter. These are brain disorders, which include delirium and dementia; psychogenic disorders, which include psychosomatic problems, neuroses, psychoses, personality problems; and learning difficulties.

Brain disorders

Brain disorders are classified as either acute or chronic. Acute brain disorders are temporary disturbances of brain function that involve a disruption of the metabolism of the brain, from which a patient usually recovers. The main symptom is often delirium; a disordered state of mind with incoherent speech, hallucinations, bewilderment, and, in its deepest stages, coma. Delirium tremens, which is suffered by alcoholics, is the best-known manifestation of an acute disorder.

Chronic brain disorders result from physical changes or damage to the tissues of the brain. Some of the damage is curable. The most common form of brain disorder is senile dementia, in which an elderly person's memory and sense of time fail progressively. Such patients need to be cared for, and medication usually cannot cure them.

Psychogenic disorders

Psychogenic disorders are defined as psychiatric conditions in which the cause of the disorder is not physical, nor is the disorder due to structural damage in the nervous system. Psychiatric disorders can produce a variety of psychiatric disturbances that range from minor to catastrophic. Some psychiatrists believe that certain psychogenic disorders are due to disturbances of the chemical balance in the nervous system.

Neuroses

Neurotic disorders are included in the psychogenic category; generally they are understandable but excessive reactions to the difficulties of living and to inner conflicts. Most people feel emotional or anxious at times, but emotions and anxiety are regarded as neurotic when they are much more intense and frequent, or last longer, than normal stress reactions. A patient needs help for a neurosis and will usually respond to treatment.

There are four main categories of neurotic disorders. They are anxiety states, reactive depression, hysterical neuroses, and obsessive or compulsive disorders. All need specific treatment.

Anxiety states can take two forms: free-floating or phobic. The first is a generalized, inexplicable feeling of dread: the sufferer cannot get to sleep or concentrate, has a pounding heart, and keeps needing to urinate. In contrast, phobic anxiety consists of feelings of panic only in certain situations—for example, in a crowd or an enclosed space. Medicines and practical techniques can be very beneficial in treating both types of anxiety.

"Reactive depression" describes the more serious aspects of feeling unhappy when something sad has happened (see Depression). If the feeling is so bad that the sufferer cannot manage ordinary activities, or if the unhappiness lasts too long, reactive depression become an illness that requires treatment.

Hysterical illnesses include physical symptoms and memory disturbances caused by anxiety. Two case studies illustrate this. The first involves a man who was angry with his unfaithful wife but was afraid that he might hit her dangerously hard. He suddenly developed a weakness in his right arm, so that he was unable to hit her. The second involves a schoolgirl who went out with a boyfriend of whom her mother disapproved. She suffered a genuine, but temporary, loss of memory, so that she did not have to explain her actions.

Obsessive or compulsive neuroses manifest themselves in the patient's inability to resist repeating certain actions, even though he or she knows that they are completely unnecessary (see Complexes and Compulsions).

Psychoses

Psychoses are psychogenic disorders in which rational thought is suspended or distorted. The patient may be unable to deal with reality and will create a private internalized environment in which his or her perceptions become delusionary or hallucinatory. The psychotic person may appear to be without emotion.

Psychoses include schizophrenia (see Schizophrenia) and bipolar disorder (see Bipolar Disorder), both of which may respond well to medication and to other forms of treatment.

Personality problems

Personality—a person's characteristic way of looking at things and of reacting to other people and situations—is unique to every human being. There are numerous distinct personality traits, and all of us have a mixture of these, with one factor predominating. One person may have a tendency to shyness, whereas another commonly has mood changes.

Personality makes people different and interesting; however, when certain traits become exaggerated they may cause problems and unhappiness. Personality characteristics seem to be emphasized when people are under stress—for instance, from physical illness or psychological strain. They can also be heightened as a result of psychiatric illness (see Personality).

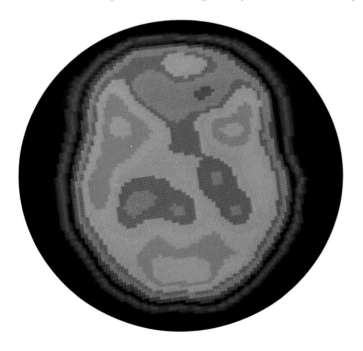
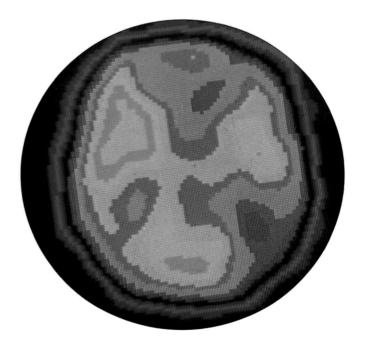

▲ *Brain scans may be used to identify areas of high metabolic activity in the brain. The patient is injected with radioactive glucose, which is absorbed by the brain cells. In* contrast to a normal scan (left), the scan of a patient in the manic phase of bipolar disorder (right) shows great activity on the right side, the red area, and an asymmetrical pattern.

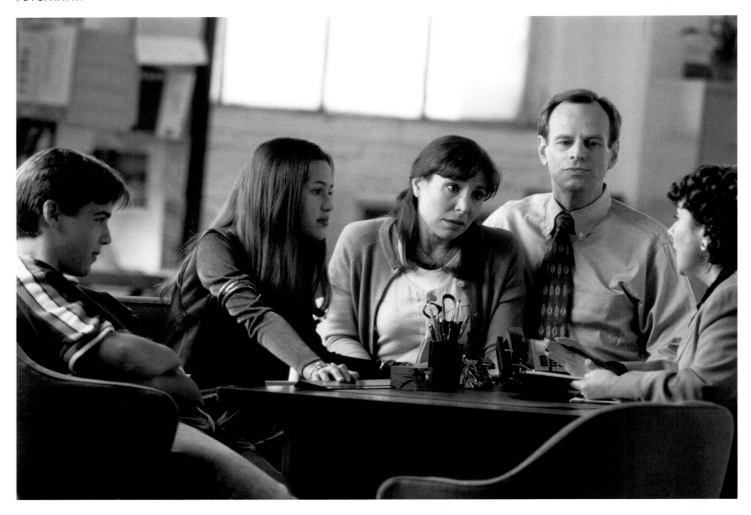

▲ *Psychiatric therapy may involve all the family. Many psychiatric problems originate because of anger or tensions, or both, in family relationships, and a frank discussion of problems can help resolve these problems.*

Psychosomatic disorders

This category of psychogenic disorder has both physical and psychiatric elements. Certain physical problems, such as ulcerative colitis, high blood pressure, and heart palpitations, are thought to have, wholly or in part, an emotional cause that results in physical or psychological changes.The term "psychosomatic" tends to be used rather loosely, and since disorders of this kind are usually marked by real physical symptoms, only a psychiatrist is qualified to judge— and even he or she may not be certain. Treatment for psychosomatic disorders will target physical and emotional sickness. If a person is suffering from a peptic ulcer which a doctor suspects is due at least in part to emotional problems, both medicines and psychological treatment may be needed (see Psychosomatic Problems).

Learning difficulties

Learning difficulties arise from faulty brain development before birth or in infancy. As a result, a young child has problems learning and may be unable to lead a normal life. Once the brain has been damaged, the condition is irreversible, but early detection and special teaching methods can minimize a child's difficulties.

Treatment in psychiatry

There is a wide variety of treatment available for psychiatric problems, ranging from group or individual therapy to different types of medication.

Psychotherapy: This is a form of treatment for emotional or psychiatric disorders through largely verbal means. All doctors talk informally when treating a patient. Formal psychotherapy, however, comes in several styles: the most simple is supportive therapy, in which the patient receives sympathy, encouragement, and appreciation to build up his or her confidence.

Another basic form of psychotherapy is insight-directed psychotherapy, in which the aim is to show the patient where he or she might have gone wrong. It also uses the technique of confrontation, or challenging the patient, to help him or her clarify actions and motives (see Psychotherapy).

Behavior therapy: In behavior therapy, the therapist tells patients directly what they must do. This is especially effective with phobic and obsessive or compulsive patients. Cognitive behavior therapy is a development in which the details of how the patient should behave are based on a study of his or her maladaptive or unhelpful beliefs and assumptions, and of negative automatic thoughts that the patient has acquired and built in as a result of early experience. Cognitive behavior therapy is empirical, structured, and educational and requires the cooperation of the patient. It is highly successful in the treatment of social phobias, shyness, obsessions, anxiety, poor self-esteem, inhibitions, poor coping skills, and many other such problems.

Psychodrama: This method helps patients understand their situation. By acting out problems, patients come to see how they may appear to other people involved. To gain an objective view, the patient takes the part of someone else.

Occupational therapy: This includes art and music therapy and is a way to help patients express their feelings, so that they can understand these feelings and gain a feeling of independence.

Medication: Although other forms of treatment play an important part in psychiatry, it is modern medication that has significantly altered the outlook for psychiatric patients, and brought psychiatric illnesses into line with treatable physical problems. Today, it is not necessary for anyone to remain in the misery of depression for months, or languish in a psychiatric unit with schizophrenia for years. Antidepressants and tranquilizers control the symptoms of many psychiatric

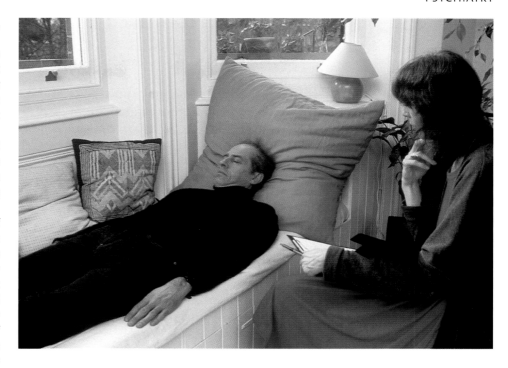

▲ *Under hypnosis, a conscious trance, a confirmed smoker can be taught to react with distaste to cigarettes.*

disorders, just as penicillin combats many physical infections. Five major types of medicine are used in treatment of psychiatric disorders today. Anxiolytics reduce tension and help the patient relax; hypnotics help a patient sleep; antipsychotics calm and clear the thinking of disturbed patients, and in small doses help combat anxiety; antidepressants help to restore a sense of hope and the ability to cope with depression; and antitension drugs release the patient—occasionally within a few days—from crippling tension which may be so severe that it involves actual physical pain.

ECT: Electroconvulsive therapy has had many frightening stories associated with it, but in cases of severe, even suicidal, depression, it may still be used. Administered by experts under the most rigidly controlled conditions, it is safe and in some circumstances acts more quickly than medication.

ECT cannot be given without signed consent, and the procedure is likely to be less unpleasant than having a tooth pulled. All that the patient is likely to remember is the injection of anesthesia.

While the patient is anesthetized a small electrical current is passed through the head for a fraction of a second: it works rather like electrical treatment for a weak muscle. Some patients experience a little difficulty in remembering minor matters from before the treatment, but this amnesia is usually only temporary.

Psychosurgery: Treatment of psychiatric disturbance by means of brain surgery, or prefrontal lobotomy, is a radical procedure, which is performed only after other forms of treatment have proved ineffective. Because of the introduction of tranquilizing drugs, there are very few cases of severe psychiatric illness that would warrant such drastic methods of treatment.

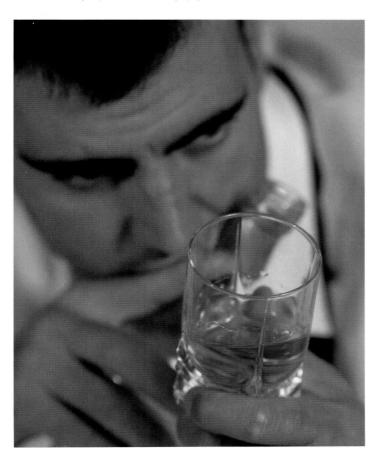

▲ *Someone addicted to alcohol can get help by attending meetings of Alcoholics Anonymous. This type of group therapy offers mutual discussion and support.*

See also: **Anxiety; Brain; Depression; Mental illness; Neuroses; Obsessive-compulsive disorder**

Psychology

Questions and Answers

Psychology means "knowledge of the mind"—how it works and why human beings and other animals think, feel, and behave the way they do. Psychologists are therefore concerned with every aspect of mental life.

People have attempted to study how the mind works for thousands of years, but it is only in the last hundred years that this study has become scientifically organized. The task is complex: at one level, the psychologist is dealing with the equivalent of a very sophisticated computer crammed into an area measuring half the size of a football; at another level the psychologist must disregard the mechanics involved and concentrate on how the person acts, thinks, and feels in an attempt to make sense of the patterns that emerge.

Because psychologists deal with all aspects of the mind, only a small part of their study deals with people's problems. In spite of this, discoveries made by psychologists may help to improve the quality of people's lives. Those who specialize in how memory works, for example, may contribute to ways of helping people whose memory is poor, and psychologists who study how we learn may be able to help us learn more easily.

Clinical psychology

Unlike the psychiatrist, who is a doctor specializing in mental health, the clinical psychologist need not have medical qualifications. However, he or she will have a degree in psychology and additional qualifications to be able to work with mental health problems.

Clinical psychologists usually work with a psychiatrist who will deal with medical matters, such as drug prescriptions. The psychologist may look after certain aspects of serious conditions such as schizophrenia and bipolar disorder, as well as less severe states such as mild depression, neuroses, and other situations that can generally be treated without the need for hospitalization (see Bipolar

What is the difference between a psychologist and a psychiatrist?

A psychiatrist is a medical doctor who specializes in the treatment of psychological mental disorders. He or she is usually attached to a hospital and may use a variety of therapeutic techniques, including drugs, to treat patients.

A psychologist will have a degree in psychology, but is usually not a medical doctor unless he or she has advanced psychological qualifications. A psychologist may advise on the working of the mind in general, but is not always a therapist: for example, he or she may specialize in social problems, clinical psychology, or education.

What practical benefit is there in understanding people's behavior?

First, we learn what behavior to expect from ourselves and others, how that behavior may change as we progress through life, and what differences we can expect between one person and another. This knowledge should make us less fearful when certain behavioral changes occur. Our understanding of patterns of behavior, thought, and feeling can also enable us to help those whose behavior is so different that it presents problems with living in society. Finally, such knowledge may keep us from labeling as "crazy" those whose ways are different from ours, yet ordinary enough to their own family or social group.

Do you have to be a doctor to give therapy or analysis?

No. Many types of therapy (of which analysis is just one) may be given by a competent psychologist. In many countries there are no laws that compel a therapist to have any qualifications, although therapists attached to a clinic or guidance center will have appropriate specialist training.

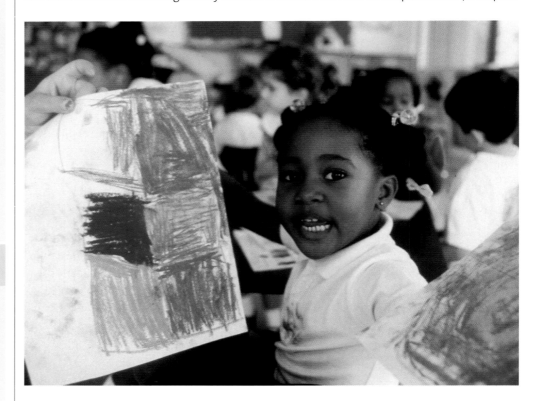

▲ *An educational psychologist often finds children's paintings helpful in assessing their motor skills and emotional state.*

Disorder; Neuroses). Clinical psychology also involves dealing with marital problems and family therapy, in which a problem may be caused not by any one person but by the relationship between two or more people.

Developmental psychology is concerned with how people change as they develop from infancy to old age. Such studies are invaluable in helping people understand what to expect at different stages in their lives, simply because they are at a given age, rather than because of any particular individual or social influences. For example, developmental psychology teaches people to expect some form of adolescent rebellion instead of being surprised or angry when it occurs (see Adolescence). Perhaps unexpectedly, it also teaches people that sexual life in late middle age is actually far more active than many people suppose. It also teaches people to accept with calmness and tolerance the slowing down of their mental processes in old age, although this may be more difficult to accept in the smaller and more self-contained families of today. This is because such families provide fewer examples of what is natural in old age than the larger, extended families of the past.

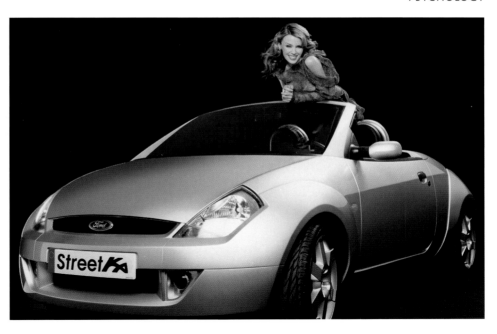

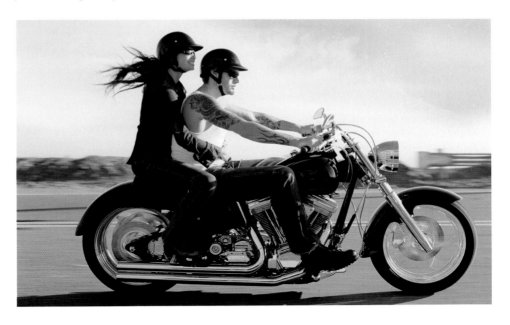

▲ ▼ *Advertisers employ sophisticated psychological techniques, whether they are trying to evoke happy, healthy family life or attempting to create a vibrant, racy, freewheeling image, as in these advertisements.*

Educational psychology

Educational psychologists deal with problems that may occur during schooling. This will involve helping young people who have a wide range of abilities, including gifted and normal children and those with learning disabilities and their parents and teachers (see Learning Disabilities). This work involves administering psychological tests, because it is sometimes possible to improve the quality of a child's education by carefully sorting out precise areas of strength and weakness and obtaining specialized help if this is necessary. For example, a child who is falling behind at school may be referred to an educational psychologist because he or she is wrongly believed to be lazy, uncaring, slow to develop, or lacking in concentration. Specialized tests may reveal, however, that the child is actually suffering from dyslexia or some other condition that involves a learning problem but does not affect the child's intelligence in any way (see Dyslexia). An educational psychologist is a specialist who tests and diagnoses conditions, devises treatment programs, and carries out treatment.

After diagnosis, the child may be referred to a therapist or some other helper. School phobia and emotional or behavioral problems may be dealt with in special classes. Sometimes, however, no referral will be necessary; a meeting with the child's teacher or the principal may be all that is needed to help steer the child toward making the best use of his or her educational abilities.

Social psychology

Social psychology is a broad field that is concerned with studying how people act in relationships with others. This encompasses how and why people form particular friendships and enmities; what the differences are in how people of different races, cultures, and classes think; the effect of changing sexual customs, violence, and the media on the way society reacts; and even the psychology of politics. All of these come under the social psychologist's scrutiny.

Although social psychology is a comparatively young branch of psychology, it is a vital part of the science, because the relationships people form with others, their society, and even with other nations will determine if and how the human species survives in the future.

Why do psychologists experiment so much on rats and pigeons?

Animal experimentation is a complex and emotional subject and one that continues to be fiercely debated. Advocates of this type of work argue that by experimenting on species with less complex brains than ours they can discover basic principles that seem also to govern the more automatic ways in which human beings tend to react to experiences.

Opponents of animal experimentation believe that, apart from any ethical considerations, the similarity between human and other animal behavior is so small that using animals in this way is worthless.

When should I expect that my child will be seen by an educational psychologist?

It is perfectly possible that your child may go through his or her formal education without ever seeing an educational psychologist. Children are generally referred only if they are having difficulty learning, or if they have a fear of going to school (school phobia) or some other behavior problem. However, if your child has seen an educational psychologist, you should not conclude that something must be wrong. A lot of research to learn about children is done using tests of one sort or another, such as those that measure intelligence, personality, and attitudes.

My nine-year-old son is a very poor reader and seems to have difficulty learning new words, even though we try to help him as much as possible at home. Should I take him to a psychologist to find out what is wrong with him?

The first thing to do, if you have not already done so, is to discuss the matter with his own teacher or with the school principal. If either thinks there is sufficient reason for it, they will refer your son to an educational psychologist for testing.

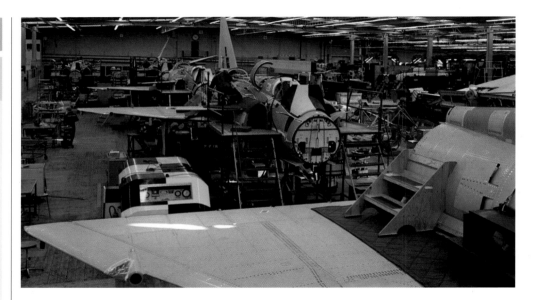

▲ *The design of a working environment—an airplane factory, for example—owes much to industrial psychology. Pleasant conditions make for more productive employees.*

Physiological psychology

Physiological psychology is the most difficult yet in some ways the most fascinating aspect of psychology. It is also the most specialized, because it is concerned with determining what parts of the brain are most involved with people's various thinking processes (see Brain). For example, physiological psychologists have discovered that certain small areas of the brain look after the activity of specific parts of the body. They have discovered that people's sense of hunger and thirst, their anger reaction, and their consciousness are all controlled and monitored by equally small brain areas, even though a memory is not located in any one particular area. The current theory of memory is that it involves active associations of groups of communicating nerve cells, gene expression, and synthesis of new proteins (see Genetics; Nervous System; Protein).

Psychologists in this field seek to find how a series of electrically charged brain cells can become the memory of a tune, an emotion, or a program for allowing a person to walk without thinking how to do it.

Industrial psychology

Although psychologists are often employed in industry, their work is usually done behind the scenes, when they are called in to advise on specific projects or aims. The training of management and other personnel can be made far more efficient by paying particular attention to such matters as people's needs, motivations, reactions, and conflicts.

Of equal importance is a clear understanding of the way people relate to each other under different circumstances, their tension and irritation, and their trust and mistrust. Psychologists are only just starting to train people to get along with one another in the workplace, although their work is more evident in salesmanship than in interactions of management and unions.

Industrial psychology also plays a part in the design of many things that people use at work. For example, the layout of an airplane instrument display panel owes much to the study of how people notice objects at the edge of their field of vision, and to the effect of looking at a complex array of slowly changing signals for long periods.

The layout of various rooms in public centers, such as hospitals, is also increasingly influenced by psychological considerations: the avoidance, when possible, of large rooms with high ceilings; the use of matte (rather than glossy) painted surfaces in varied colors; the use of pictures, photographs, and ornaments; the availability of private areas; and generally the opportunity for patients to express their individuality. Some or all of these factors may help to speed up the recovery of a patient who is receiving treatment in the hospital.

See also: Depression; Family relationships; Memory; Mental illness; Mind; Phobias; Psychiatry; Schizophrenia; Therapy

Psychoses

Questions and Answers

My brother is seventeen. He has told me that for several months he has been in almost daily contact with a spirit guide who is now running his life. This guide appears to him nearly every night and tells him many things including how he is to protect himself from the enemy's atomic radiation. Is this serious?

Regrettably, it probably is. Your brother should be seen by a psychiatrist without delay.

My 82-year-old mother has become very confused and disoriented in recent months. She is inclined to wander off on her own, sometimes only partly dressed, and often can't find her way home and has to be brought back by the police. Is she suffering from a psychosis?

Probably not. There is a difference between a severe disorder of mind, which may be a psychosis, and severe loss of mind, which is called dementia. It's not possible from your description to be sure what is wrong with your mother, but it is obvious that she urgently needs expert medical and psychiatric evaluation. She may be developing Alzheimer's disease or another form of dementia. She may have a treatable organic disorder that imitates dementia. A small proportion of older people who appear demented can actually be restored to normal by medical treatment.

My husband died a year ago and since then, on four occasions, I'm sure I saw him. I have also heard him talk to me. I'm afraid I am going mad. Is this a psychosis?

No. It is common for a bereaved person to believe the deceased person is present and is speaking. Although this is a hallucination it is an entirely normal experience and there is no need to worry.

Psychoses are major psychiatric disorders and are a cause of enormous suffering both to those affected and to their families and friends. Psychotic disorders disrupt lives and seriously interfere with human relationships.

The basic difference between a psychosis and any other form of psychiatric disorder is that a psychotic person has, to a greater or lesser extent, lost contact with reality. Such a person also has various convictions and experiences that differ so markedly from those of most people that they are generally considered unbelievable. These two patterns of experience are summed up in the terms "delusions" and "hallucinations."

Psychotic or normal?

A person who has delusions and hallucinations is not necessarily psychotic. Most people have delusions, usually because of misinterpretation of received information, and many people have hallucinations from time to time. Psychotic delusions and hallucinations are, however, quite different from these normal patterns. People with an acute psychotic disorder are so affected by distortion or disorganization of thought, emotion, and grasp of reality that they are incapable of relating normally to other people or coping with the demands of everyday life. They are totally unaware that there is anything wrong with their beliefs and perceptions. In medical terms, such people have no insight into their condition.

Because delusions and hallucinations are very real to them, they will often react in a manner that would be sensible and rational if the delusions and hallucinations were really true. This is why psychotic people are often violent or agitated or are capable of extreme behavior, and sometimes even of violence or homicide.

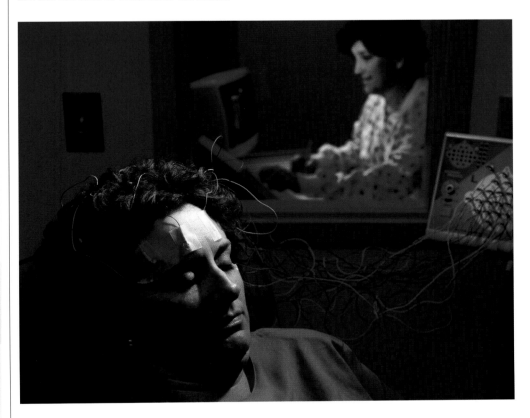

▲ *In cases of psychotic disorder, a brain function test, such as an electroencephalograph (EEG), is just one of the diagnostic tools available.*

My cousin has bipolar disorder and has started taking lithium. The drug disagrees with her; she feels nauseated and shaky and is always thirsty. Should she stop taking it?

Certainly not before discussing the side effects with her doctor, who will carry out tests to measure the drug levels. Lithium is a mood-stabilizing drug and can control the symptoms of bipolar disorder. At first, many people who take lithium experience these side effects, but as treatment is continued, they do lessen in severity. Your cousin should make certain she never gets dehydrated, and does not alter the amount of salt that she eats with her food, since these factors can affect the levels of lithium in the body.

What is the outlook for someone who has schizophrenia?

Schizophrenia generally is a long-term illness, but about 20 percent of people have one episode, which never recurs, and they continue to have a normal life. For the remaining 80 percent, the illness is characterized by many episodes, which have severe symptoms. Patients will usually have to stay in the hospital after one of these episodes, and when they are discharged they will need support and care. If the disorder starts at an early age, the long-term outlook is not so good.

Do antipsychotic drugs have side effects, and how do they work?

Yes. These drugs can lower blood pressure, causing dizziness, blurred vision, and a dry mouth. The side effects lessen with time, but after lengthy use, jerking movements of the face and mouth become permanent.

Antipsychotic drugs work by blocking a brain chemical called dopamine. The chemical, which is present in high amounts in psychotic disorders, is thought to cause the symptoms.

Some antipsychotic drugs block other chemicals that can alter a person's mood.

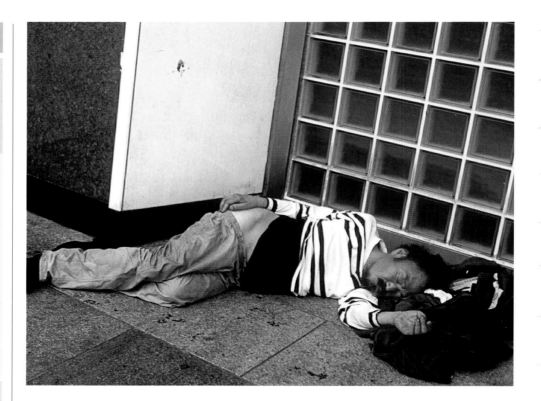

▲ *Many homeless people who live on the streets are suffering from a psychotic disorder, such as schizophrenia, which causes an inability to function socially.*

Psychotic delusions

Delusions are fixed beliefs in the reality of something that is manifestly absurd or untrue. It is not always easy to distinguish psychotic delusions from a rigidly held but mistaken conviction, but most of them are so inherently improbable, or so obviously based on faulty perceptions or reasoning, that they clearly indicate serious mental disturbance.

Paranoid delusions

One form of psychotic delusion is an unjustified conviction of being persecuted. This is called a paranoid delusion. Delusions of persecution vary considerably in detail but will always relate to some hostile external agency that means harm. It is common for the sufferer to be convinced that this outside agency is controlling his or her thoughts, actions, moods, emotions or state of health. In order to make sense of the situation some kind of explanation has to be developed, and this will be influenced by what the patient already knows. For this reason, historically, there have seemed to be fashions in psychotic delusions that fitted in with advances in scientific knowledge.

Other delusions

Psychotic delusions are not all delusions of persecution. Other common delusions include delusions of grandeur in which the affected person is convinced of having a social, financial, educational, or political status that is much higher than reality; hypochondriacal delusions of serious illness involving internal rotting or other improbable bodily effects; delusions of severe abnormality of body shape that is, however, imperceptible to others; convictions that the sufferer is, in fact, another, and usually famous, person; feelings that mundane objects have a great significance; and delusions of personal unworthiness.

Psychotic delusions are often part of a systematized and coherent rationalization. A psychotic patient might, for instance, believe that although he is a member of a very distinguished and wealthy family, possibly with a European royal title, it is essential, for political reasons, or for the sake of security, for this fact to be concealed.

Systematized delusions are characteristic of schizophrenia and often have an internal logic that could not be faulted if one accepted the premises on which they are based. Delusions of

the production of high blood pressure. When any animal, including a human being, prepares to deal with an external emergency, one of the many physical changes that are required is increased circulatory effort. To bring this about, the heart is stimulated to beat more powerfully and faster, and blood pressure is increased. When the emergency is over, the blood pressure returns to its normal level. If, however, the blood pressure is raised repeatedly, perhaps continually, as a response to some emotional stress, secondary changes take place in the blood vessels and in the kidneys and brain so that permanent damage to these structures may result (see Blood Pressure; Stress).

Studies show that in only 1 or 2 percent of patients with severely raised blood pressure is there any other pathological cause for the condition.

It is not only anxiety that can be accompanied by body changes and symptoms. Other strong feelings such as anger, frustration, and guilt as well as stress can also be accompanied by symptoms.

Diagnosis

When patients consult a doctor about any symptoms or illness, it is always of great help for him or her to know about any important life changes, or about any recent emotional upsets or problems. Once a doctor has taken a full history of symptoms and how they occurred, a tentative diagnosis can be made. A physical examination is frequently required only to confirm what has emerged from the history.

It is not enough to exclude the presence of physical disease, and then to diagnose an illness caused mainly by an emotional problem. This diagnosis must be made on positive evidence of some actual emotional difficulty that can then be fully explored. If in spite of a thorough discussion between doctor and patient there is no apparent emotional cause, the diagnosis must be reconsidered. However, it must be remembered that on occasions the emotional content may be repressed, either because the patient has subconsciously dismissed it or because it is not in the conscious memory. In such cases, only further discussion, perhaps in psychotherapy, will help to identify the problem.

Treatment

Many psychosomatic illnesses can be treated in a doctor's office, provided that the patient feels able to talk to his or her doctor and

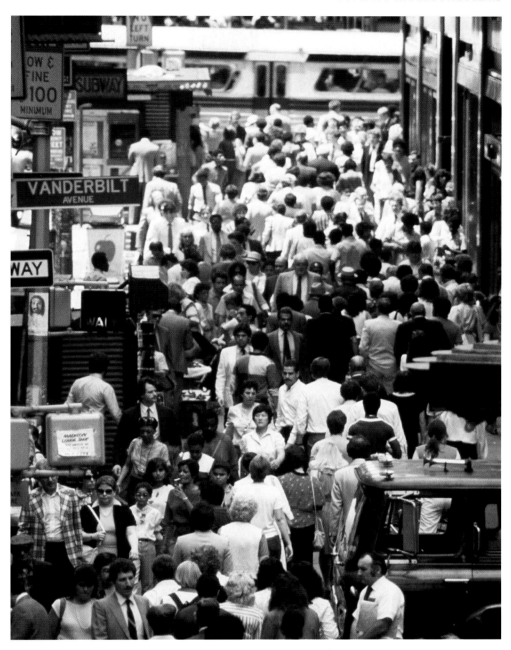

▲ *Overcrowding on the streets and subways as well as other daily stresses can lead to physical damage if the stress is prolonged.*

that the doctor has the time to listen. Although it is not the doctor's job to tell patients how to live their lives, it is nevertheless helpful for the doctor to guide them in a direction that appears to be useful in alleviating the problem.

Feelings of tension experienced by a patient can also be reduced by a certain amount of emotional reeducation. Methods of dealing with a problem, whether it is a difficult personal relationship or a problem at work, might be discovered by the patient and the doctor, or by a health professional, such as a psychologist or therapist. Exercise, relaxation, and therapies to reduce stress may also prove helpful.

See also: **Asthma; Coronary arteries and thrombosis**

INDEX